A Change of Mind

One family's journey through brain injury

Janelle Breese Biagioni

Cover photo courtesy of Robert Mullin, Penticton Herald

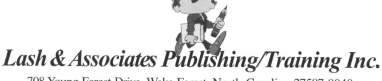

Lash & Associates Publishing/Training Inc.

708 Young Forest Drive, Wake Forest, North Carolina 27587-9040

First Edition

This publication is sold with the understanding that the publisher is not engaged in rendering legal, financial, medical, or other such services. If legal or other expert assistance is required, a competent professional in the appropriate field should be sought. All brand and product names are trademarks or registered trademarks of their respective companies.

Published by Lash & Associates Publishing/Training Inc., 708 Young Forest Drive, Wake Forest, NC 27587 Tel: & Fax: (919) 562-0015

You may order this book directly from the publisher by calling (919) 562-0015 or visiting our website at www.lapublishing.com

Library of Congress Control Number: 2004100681

ISBN 1931117197-5

Table of Contents

Introduction

The siren screamed as metal twisted, scraping and gouging the rough pavement.

The overturned police bike spun in circles, imbedding streaks of blue and white paint into the asphalt road.

The loaded .38 revolver flew from the officer's holster as his body hurled through the air.

The force of his feet smashing against the side of the car catapulted him over the roof.

His portable radio separated from the belt and broke through the car's passenger window, viciously striking the 74-year-old woman driver.

As the officer's body landed with a thud face down on the pavement, the base of his right thumb shattered and the layers of skin exposed beneath his short sleeves peeled away.

Skidding sideways, his forehead crashed against the cement curb cracking his protective helmet.

The weight of his body flipped him over, crunching his face into the stop sign, breaking his nose and splitting his lips and chin in half.

Blood gushed from his face as his limp body came to rest on his back on the sidewalk.

Pooling in his mouth, the blood congealed at the back of his throat.

He began to choke.

His airway closed, thrusting him into full cardiac arrest.

Suddenly, the world stopped. His world – my world...

The Long Weekend

It was shortly after 8:00 p.m. on May 19, 1990 and the start of a busy long weekend in Penticton, British Columbia. My husband, Gerry Breese, a constable for 17 years in the Royal Canadian Mounted Police (RCMP), had just begun the second of three night shifts. On that particular morning, I woke feeling rested and unsuspecting that life was about to change. For the past year, I had been studying the Certified General Accountants' course by correspondence. Each weekly lesson required about 15-20 hours of study time and included an assignment that had to be postmarked by Saturday morning. I was one day ahead of schedule, so I planned to take the day off to accomplish some late spring-cleaning. As a reward for helping with what we referred to as "the de-munging" of their bedrooms, I promised our daughters, Myriah age 12, and Dale age 10, that I would take them into town to visit friends for the evening while their Dad was working.

We lived in the quaint village of Naramata, British Columbia, with a population of less than two thousand. The village is approximately thirteen miles north of the city of Penticton, B.C., a Canadian resort area known for its semi-arid climate and beautiful lakes. Our home, situated on a small parcel of land, overlooked a creek in the back and faced an apple orchard in the front. That morning the valley was drenched in sunshine. The refreshing spring air and soothing sounds of chirping birds commanded windows and doors be opened to allow nature's beauty to be seen, felt and heard.

Around 4:30 p.m., Gerry stumbled down the stairs into the kitchen not at all looking like he wanted to work another graveyard shift. His thick dirty-blond hair was tousled and his crystal blue eyes reddened from lack of sleep. I silently sympathized, as his five-foot ten-inch, 200-pound frame staggered toward the table while he casually scratched his belly. In his hand was a pager, which kept him abreast of activity at Naramata's fire hall. Being a volunteer fireman often conflicted with his work schedule as a police officer. However, he believed it was his contribution to our local community, one he was proud of, even though it left him with little sleep on weekends like this.

Gerry tucked the pager into the charger on the counter before sitting down at the table. He leisurely leaned back in the chair, stretching his legs, letting out a ferocious yawn. His mouth gaped while he vigorously rubbed his eyes to clear the cobwebs.

"Shit!" he blurted, bolting his body upright and propping his elbows on the table.

I handed him a cup of hot coffee.

"Good morning," he grunted.

"Good afternoon," I corrected, before kissing his cheek. "Did you have a good sleep?"

"Not bad."

"I hope we didn't make too much noise."

"Nope. Where are the kids?"

"Downstairs, watching TV. They really worked hard around here today."

Gerry's face reddened from coughing as he lit a filtered cigarette; a habit he'd had since the age of fourteen. He quickly took another puff, glancing around the open kitchen.

"Yeah – it looks good in here."

"Well, I feel better," I replied, "but I still need to scrub walls." Teasingly, I added, "You know, I love the wood heater you put in, but let met tell you, it leaves dust and cobwebs everywhere."

Wood had been the main source of heat for him as a child growing up in northern British Columbia. The sound of apple wood crackling in the heater created a sense of home to him. And I can't say it didn't intoxicate me with the same warmth.

"Are you studying tonight?" he asked, glancing at the stack of textbooks on the kitchen floor.

"No. Thank heavens! My assignment went in the mail last night. I've decided to take the night off and go into town with the kids."

A Change of Mind

"Good. What are you going to do?"

"We're going over to the Ogdens. Ruth, Heather, Becky, the girls and I are going to the rock and gem show near their house. Dale really wants to see it. It's free and I thought it would be kind of fun. What do you think?"

"I think it's a great idea. Just be careful though. There are a lot of assholes on the street this weekend."

The imitation brass wall clock in the living room suddenly chimed. I took the ding-dong as my cue to start dinner. As I took my place at the cooking island in the center of our recently renovated kitchen and opened a package of waiting spareribs, I asked Gerry about his shift the night before.

Much like Fort Lauderdale, our community swells by the thousands on long weekends, creating a tremendous amount of work for the local police with many complaints of loud parties, drinking-related assaults and major traffic snarls.

"Oh, just the usual," he replied, jumping up from his chair. "It's okay for me, but I want you guys to be careful." He stood behind me playfully wrapping his arms around my waist and nuzzling my neck.

"Where's my kidlets? I haven't seen them since yesterday."

"Downstairs, for the second time."

"Right! I'll go say hello and then jump in the shower. As soon as I'm done, I'll throw those ribs on the barbecue."

He dashed down the newly carpeted basement stairs in search of our daughters, ignoring the ringing telephone as he passed it. I shook my head, wishing that I could ignore it too. Instead, I wiped my greasy hands on a kitchen towel and reached for the receiver.

"Hello?"

"Hi Janelle. It's Ruth."

"Hi Ruth. How are you?"

"Well, it's been one of those days."

"Uh, oh … what's wrong?"

"Nothing really. Just the usual…" she said, her voice trailing in despair.

Ruth Ogden was one of my closest friends and her husband, Bob, was Gerry's shift boss. Three years earlier, Bob and Ruth had been transferred to the Penticton Detachment. My friendship with Ruth was concrete from the moment she and I met. She was very down-to-earth and easy to be with. Bob and Ruth had two daughters, fairly close in age to our girls.

Tragedy had struck only a few months after the Ogden's arrived in Penticton. While crossing at a crosswalk on their way to a Saturday afternoon matinee, Ruth and her daughter Becky were hit by a car. Becky was uninjured, but Ruth had suffered a severe brain injury and sustained permanent brain damage. While Ruth had made tremendous strides in regaining control of her life, she had permanent deficits with losses in short-term memory, speech and hearing, and her sense of taste and smell. She had great difficulty with abstract thinking. Because of these losses, she was unable to return to work outside her home and this devastated her.

The bond between us got even stronger after her accident. We were steadfast in working through her accomplishments and disappointments together. This was not to say that our relationship didn't undergo some changes. It did. And some of these changes were significant.

Our friendship evolved from an equal partnership of give and take, to one where I played the role of mother, caregiver, and big sister as Ruth strived to regain control of her life. At times, I resented (guiltily) these changes, feeling very sad about "letting go" of the Ruth I once knew. Nonetheless, she remained one of my best friends, offering me new challenges and teaching me valuable lessons on preserving the dignity of living with a disability. These were lessons that could only be learned from first-hand experience as I found out for myself later.

A Change of Mind

Ruth's silence on the other end of the phone evoked my usual response as I automatically offered a sympathetic ear. "That's too bad. Are you still feeling up to going out tonight?"

"Yeah. That's why I called… to see if you're still coming into town."

"You bet. I'll be at your place by seven o'clock. We might as well walk from your house to the rock and gem show. You can tell me all about your day then."

"Okay," Ruth replied. "That sounds good. I'll see you then."

After hanging up the telephone I looked up to see Gerry standing by the stove. Freshly showered, his wet hair was uncombed and stood up in spots. He resembled a little boy as tiny water droplets dripped down his baby face to his neck, finally coming to rest on his bare shoulders.

"Who was that?" he asked, curiously.

"Ruth."

"How is she?"

"Sounds like she had a bad day so I'll see if we can't cheer her up tonight."

I walked over and wrapped my arms around his neck and looked lovingly into his eyes. He responded by kissing me lightly on the nose. I couldn't help thinking how lucky I was. Quietly, I said, "I don't know what I'd do if something ever happened to you."

Gerry flashed a smile exposing his perfectly straight white teeth as he nudged my chin with a crooked finger. "Nothing's going to happen to me. Don't let it get to you."

I knew he was right, but the fear of something happening at work was something a police officer's spouse lived with everyday. It's always tucked away in the back of your mind ready to spring forward at the slightest touch like a "jack in the box".

A Change of Mind

The Crash

The second hand on the kitchen clock ticked steadily after dinner, keeping us on schedule. Gerry soon stood at the front door and said goodbye. I watched him swing his leg over his Kawasaki motorcycle, a Father's Day gift the year before, and slam his cowboy boot down hard to kick-start the motor. In an exaggerated motion, he tipped a hand from the peak of his helmet to salute me. He guided the bike slowly down the driveway and shouted over the revving motor, "See you in the morning."

With my hands on each child's shoulder, I gently steered them towards our station wagon. Myriah, our eldest and most practical daughter, stuck out her lower lip and defiantly kicked the toe of her running shoe into the gravel. "I wanted to ride on the bike with Dad."

"Not tonight, Honey. Maybe Daddy can take you for a ride tomorrow. Come on now. We're in a bit of a hurry to get to Ruth's."

Later that night, I learned Gerry had arrived at the office and in his usual boyish manner, took time to joke with fellow police officers, the office staff, and the radio dispatcher. My younger brother, Nathan Davies was also there because he worked as a part-time guard in the city jail, located in the basement of the police detachment.

Shortly after their shift started, several officers responded to an alleged stabbing in the south end of town. True to his nature, Gerry responded to their call for back up, even though his immediate duties as a motorcycle officer revolved around city traffic. Eyewitnesses who were interviewed that night reported seeing Gerry stopped at a red light and speaking into the radio microphone that was attached to his shirt collar. They watched him flick on the bike's red flashing light before cautiously turning left to travel south in the left lane of a one-way street. One block away, an elderly woman who had just finished working at a wedding reception eased her car away from the curb. Apparently, she didn't see the police bike approaching from behind and continued across two lanes to turn onto a side street. As best as the investigators can figure, it seemed Gerry changed lanes to try to avoid her. Seconds later, all our lives changed forever. Bystanders screamed as vehicles screeched to a stop. Drivers and passengers jumped out of their vehicles for a better view. One split second of error and strangers on the sidewalk were praying for Gerry's survival. An off-duty Vancouver City police officer was one of the drivers who stopped to help. Hurrying from his car, he ran to Gerry's gun that lay on the road in open view. By taking it into his possession, the officer ensured that the gun did not land in the hands of an irresponsible person. A woman on the sidewalk shouted she would go get her brother, a trained paramedic who lived nearby.

Jake Wiens, a local cab driver trained in first-aid, stopped his car to see if he could help. To his horror, the seemingly lifeless victim was the police officer he had passed only minutes earlier. He placed a call to the taxicab dispatcher to notify the RCMP that one of their officers was down and that an ambulance was needed.

Minutes earlier, the police dispatcher had asked Nathan to come up from the jail to answer the phones and radio for him while he took his supper break. "I'll be back in half an hour, Nathan. The boys are going to a call on the south side of town. Everything else is quiet," advised the dispatcher.

Nathan fell into a chair, sliding it across the floor to stop at the desk where the telephone and radio were. "No problem. Take your time."

The telephone rang as the dispatcher picked his car keys up from the counter. "Damn it. Just when you think it's quiet!"

Nathan waved a hand, dismissing the hungry young man. "Forget it. Go on. I'll take it."

Nathan tucked the mouthpiece under his chin and routinely grasped a pen to make notes. "Penticton, RCMP. Davies speaking."

"This is the cab company. There's been an accident." the caller blurted. "It's one of your police officers... the one on the motorcycle...he's been hit by a car!"

The muscles in Nathan's back tightened. He moved the phone to his other ear as if it would change what he was hearing.

"The policeman on the motorcycle is injured. He needs an ambulance right away."

Nathan's heart pounded as he struggled to maintain some professionalism, knowing the female caller was talking about his brother-in-law. Covering the mouthpiece, he shouted for Cy Kelly, the shift corporal.

"Cy, get in here! Breese has been hit by a car..."

"Excuse me ... Hello? Are you there?" questioned the woman waiting on the phone.

"Sorry Ma'am. Yes, I'm here. Can you tell me where the accident is?"

"At the corner of Martin Street and Orchard Avenue. One of our drivers is there now. He knows first-aid, but he needs an ambulance."

"Okay, Ma'am. Thanks for calling. We're on our way."

"What's going on Nathan?" Corporal Kelly was now standing on the other side of the counter.

Nathan referred to his brother-in-law by his nickname. "Mad Dog's been hit on the bike. Call an ambulance. He's at Orchard and Martin. I have to try and find my sister."

The telephone lines lit up in unison. Nathan cut off the next caller. "We already have the call, sir. An ambulance is on the way."

Nathan slammed down the phone. "You got that ambulance yet, Cy?" He waved with one hand, indicating it was done.

In the next room, Cy Kelly jumped up from his chair pulling truck keys from his pocket. Not wasting one precious moment, he brushed past the steno and dispatcher who were returning from their break, telling them about Gerry's accident using the bike's code name. "Charlie-1's been hit! Help Nathan find his wife so we can dispatch someone to get her."

The dispatcher halted abruptly and looked at the steno whose color had suddenly drained from her cheeks. "Oh my God! That's

Gerry! How bad is he hurt, Cy?"

Cy rushed past the radio room, hollering, "It looks bad."

The dispatcher hurried into the radio room and picked up the call sheet to scan Nathan's notes. He sat down next to the large tape recorder used in recording calls as they came in, and carefully listened to Nathan's telephone conversation.

"Yes, sir... we received the call about the party. We'll send a car as soon as we can. All our members are tied up right now!" Smashing down the phone, Nathan reached over the desk and snapped the music off, pounding a fist on the counter. "Damn it!"

The steno entered the radio room with fresh cups of coffee, but the phone system lit up again before Nathan could take his cup. At the same time, a voice blasted over the radio. The dispatcher answered the phone. Nathan took the call on the radio. It was Cy Kelly, who had left the office just minutes earlier.

"Penticton-Echo 4. Where the fuck is that ambulance?" Cy's voice was tense.

"I'll phone right away Cy and find out where the hell they are."

In the meantime, Corporal Kelly arrived at the accident scene where chaos seemed to prevail. He pushed his way through the crowd on the sidewalk. Jake Wiens, the cab driver, and Jeff Nielson, the brother of the bystander who had run three blocks to get him, were hunched over Gerry.

Jake, the cab driver had been the first to arrive. Jeff and his wife Louise had been unpacking moving crates when his sister burst through the door pleading for his help. Without hesitation, Jeff immediately stopped what he was doing and followed his sister out the door. Running down the front stairs of the house, he shouted for his wife to find his medical bag and follow him. The brother and sister team ran down the street and around the corner. Politely pushing his way through the onlookers, Jeff dropped to his knees beside the officer. He briefly acknowledged Jake, who was crouched across from him and unbuttoning Gerry's bloodstained shirt.

"Hi. I'm Jeff – a paramedic – we just moved here from Alberta."

"Jake," was all the other man said.

Jeff checked Gerry's wrist for a pulse first before placing two fingers on the side of his neck. Nothing! "I can't locate a pulse," Jeff flashed at Jake. "You check. If you can't find anything, I'll start CPR."

Jake placed his fingers on the identical spots with the same results as Jeff. Working quickly, they tilted Gerry's blood-soaked head upwards, applying pressure to open his mouth. Sliding his fingers inside Gerry's mangled mouth, Jeff probed for the obstruction that blocked his airway. Scooping with two fingers, he dislodged a blood clot the size of a man's fist. After following all the necessary procedures, Jeff clasped his hands - one over the back of the other - on Gerry's chest to begin compressions.

"One... two... three..."

Beads of sweat trickled down his temple and under the frames of his eyeglasses, landing on his cheek. Tossing his head back to search the crowd, he called to the uniformed police officer standing nearby. "Where's that ambulance? We need help!"

Cy slid his portable radio from his hip and called into the Penticton office, "Call the fucking dispatch for the ambulance and find out where it is."

Nathan reached for the phone as he listened intently to the noise on the radio. He heard Cy's voice crack in the background.

"We're losing him boys. We need some help!"

Nathan's voice quivered as he spoke into the microphone. "Cy...Cy...Hang in there, big guy. The ambulance was tied up with the stabbing, but they're on their way."

Cy quickly replied: "Yeah, yeah … they're here now. The ambulance has arrived!"

Nathan could hear the eerie shrill of the ambulance's siren in the background. He leaned forward, placing his elbows on the desk and resting his forehead on the tips of his fingers. The minute hand on the wall clock moved slowly. The silence was painful. Slapping his palm flat on the countertop, Nathan bellowed into the microphone: "Damn it! Somebody say something!"

Meanwhile, off-duty police officers and office staff gathered silently outside the radio room to listen to the incoming radio calls. Goosebumps crept up Nathan's arms when he heard the sound of people cheering over the microphone. "What's going on Cy?"

"They have a pulse...oh, God...they did it. They have a pulse!" screamed Cy.

Nathan rushed to the doorway where the small crowd was hugging one another. The dispatcher grasped Nathan's hand and shook it hard. "Yahoo! He's alive! All right!" Nathan squealed, releasing the dispatcher's hand so he could wrap his arms around the man's broad shoulders. The radio crackled. Nathan gave one final shout before lifting the microphone to answer. "Penticton-Bravo 1."

The new voice was Corporal Bob Ogden. He had just come from the stabbing call. "Bravo 1-Penticton."

"Yeah, Nathan. I'm clear. How's Mad Dog?

"He's in tough shape, Oggie. They've transported him to the hospital. I'm about to send a car to Naramata to pick up Janelle."

"Never mind. She's at my house visiting Ruth. I've sent Amelia to get her. I'm heading to the hospital right now."

"10-4. I'll be there as soon as I can get someone to relieve me," replied Nathan.

The hospital parking lot began to fill with marked and unmarked cruisers. The sidewalk was lined with police officers and emergency department staff awaiting the arrival of the ambulance. Peter Quandt, a handsome man and our family doctor, who possesses all the endearing qualities of a country doctor, happened to be the physician on call. He instinctively knew it was Gerry when he received the call. Dr. Quandt, who also lived in Naramata, later told me that Gerry had been traveling right behind him into town that night and that Gerry eventually passed Quandt with a nod and a wave.

Ears perked and feet began to shuffle as the ambulance came into view, siren blaring and lights flashing. The man driving the ambulance pushed the gearshift into park and threw open his door, running to the back of the vehicle to open its double doors. Another attendant along with Jake Wiens and Jeff Nielson climbed out, sliding the blood-splattered gurney with them.

The men dropped the wheels with a snap, locked them into position and rapidly wheeled the stretcher toward the emergency doors. Gerry's teeth clenched the tube that had been inserted into his mouth to keep the airway open. Gurgling and moaning with excruciating pain, he drifted in and out of consciousness.

The entourage of uniformed officers closed in, blocking any view of the emergency room. Dr. Quandt's orders to take him up to Intensive Care rang through the night air as the glass doors swished shut.

My Worst Fear

At 9:00 p.m., Bob Ogden dispatched Amelia Hayden to his home. The blue and red flashing lights on her police car peaked the curiosity of dog walkers, bicyclers, and couples perched on front porches enjoying the mild evening air. Unsuspecting, Ruth and I had just returned from the rock and gem show with our daughters. We sat on matching love seats, sipping iced soft drinks and enjoying the quiet. Classical music played softly in the background. All four daughters had retreated to the lower level of the house with a supply of pop and chips to listen to the latest rock tape.

Remembering how depressed Ruth had sounded, I eased into the topic of her health, knowing she would confide in me. "Have you got the results of your tests back?"

"Yeah, yesterday. They couldn't find anything."

Immediately I understood the reason behind Ruth's depression. She had begun having seizures over the past month, often with no warning, causing tremendous embarrassment. Since her brain injury, she'd been through a frustrating series of ups and downs and the only answer she seemed to get from the doctors was, "Wait and see." She had hoped this time would be different and she would get some concrete answers.

"Nothing?" I questioned, almost disbelieving. "What are the seizures from then?"

"My brain injury. The doctor said it often happens a couple of years after."

"Is there anything they can do for them?"

"They gave me some pills to take everyday. They said that should control them."

I sensed some resentment in Ruth's voice.

"I'm just so fed up with it. All the doctors say that I have to learn to live with these things." Ruth hesitated momentarily. "That's fine for them - it's not their life."

I nodded as Ruth went on to say, "It's just like the insurance company. I can never get a straight answer from them. Janelle, I hope you never have to deal with them because it's just awful!"

The thickly folded sheer curtains on the living room window and the tall trees in the front yard prevented us from seeing the police car turning into the cul de sac. Normally, the arrival of a police car at the Ogden house wouldn't attract attention, but tonight was different. The flashing lights were a sign that this was more than a social call. Gathering at the edge of their lawns, several neighbors watched curiously as the lights turned off and two officers stepped out of the car.

Heather, age 15, had just returned from the kitchen with drink refills. The suddenness of the doorbell startled us.

"I'll get it, Mom," called Heather from around the corner.

We could hear muffled voices outside. Ruth edged forward on the love seat, straining to hear the conversation. Heather stepped outside, closing the door quietly behind her.

"It must be one of Heather's friends," I said.

"Heather would have told me who was here," Ruth replied, matter-of-factly.

My curiosity began to stir, edging me forward on the love seat. Ruth and I studied each other's faces as we waited. After a few seconds we headed for the window to see who Heather was talking to. By slightly moving the curtains, we could see a police car parked in the driveway, but trees and a corner of the house blocked our view. Reacting as though we were suddenly invading someone's privacy, Ruth and I dropped the curtains and quickly returned to our seats. Instinct told me something was wrong.

From the lack of color in Ruth's face and the tremble of her hand, I knew she felt the same.

Gerry and I had been married fourteen years. Bob and Ruth had been married for nearly twenty. The fear of something happening to our husbands while they were on duty had always been in the back of our minds. But never, ever, in my wildest dreams had I felt the ominous threat of danger, as I did then. It never occurred to me that the call might be for Ruth. Paralyzed with fear, I clenched my hands on my lap, never taking my eyes off her. The wait seemed endless.

"I can't stand this," Ruth said. "I have to see what's going on."

My eyes followed her as she descended down the short flight of stairs to the front door. I listened as the door opened and then closed. My hands were tucked under my thighs and I nervously tapped my feet. Moments later the door opened and I walked to the stairs, expecting to see Ruth. However, I was surprised to meet Heather instead, her green eyes wide.

"You can't go out there right now, Mrs. Breese. My Mom will be back in a minute," she instructed, dashing through the laundry room in an effort to avoid further conversation with me.

"Oh, my God! This is it! I know it's bad news." I said to myself. Folding my hands over my stomach, I breathed quickly. My heart pounded. I breathed faster and faster, until finally dizziness forced me to return to the love seat and sit with my head between my knees.

"This is crazy – I don't even know what's going on," I said bolting upright, my words echoing in the empty room. The sound of the front door brought me to my feet. Moving quickly to the top of the stairs, I saw Constable Amelia Hayden. Her ashen face and reddened eyes confirmed my deepest fear. Clipping her portable radio on to her holster, she kept her eyes fixed on mine as she climbed to the top step. I wanted to run, to escape, as though I were a fugitive backed into a corner. I turned away from her, but there was nowhere to go. My knees wobbled and my hands began to sweat. Twisting my body around, I faced her.

"Maybe you'd like to have a seat, Janelle," she said, more in the way of an order.

I used one hand to wipe the perspiration from my upper lip, pressing the other hand firmly into my stomach, fighting a wave of nausea. "God, no, Amelia. Just tell me what happened."

My eyes bounced from Amelia to Ruth, hoping. Amelia's black boot hit the tip of my toes as she stopped and firmly gripped my arm.

"Gerry's been in a very bad accident. He's alive, but he's in serious condition. The ambulance should be at the hospital right now."

My eyes stung. "What happened, Amelia?"

"I don't know all the details," she replied. "I only know he was on the police motorcycle and was hit by a car. Bob is waiting at the hospital for you. He'll give you all the details." Wrapping her arms around me, she whispered in a strained voice, "I'm so sorry. Hang in there. I'll take you right to him."

Ruth stood still, almost like a statue, appearing unshaken by the news. Although I was panic stricken, I remember being surprised by her stoic response. Knowing just how difficult it was for her to cope with stressful situations since her accident, this was completely uncharacteristic for her.

"Oh, Ruth, this is the last thing you need." I said automatically as I rushed to her.

"It's okay, Janelle. You go to the hospital. I'll take care of the girls. Don't even say good-bye to them. I'll explain that you'll come back as soon as you know what's going on." We hugged and Ruth continued to offer encouragement. "Now don't worry. Gerry's a fighter. I know he's going to make it!"

I nodded as Ruth let go of me, and I headed to the door, stopping only to pick up my shoes and purse. I tucked them under my arm and ran to the police car, feeling my heart pounding in my chest with every step.

As quickly and skillfully as Amelia drove the police car, my mind willed it to go faster. Covering my whitened knuckles with her hand, Amelia told me Bob's instructions were for her to notify family and pick up anyone needing a ride to the hospital. I used the sleeve of my sweatshirt to dry my eyes. The list of the people raced through my mind.

"Oh, God, I can hardly think, Amelia. Someone needs to call

Nathan and get him to get a hold of my Mom."

"Nathan's working at the police station," Amelia replied.

"He'll be meeting you at the hospital, but I can get your Mom. What's her address?"

"Uh...uh...9...934 Killarney. Right on the corner of Forestbrook and Killarney."

"Okay, I'll drop you off and then go pick her up. Anyone else?"

"No, I don't think so. Thanks...Mom and Nathan will call everybody else."

My throat felt dry. My eyes burned. "This can't be happening! I just don't believe it," I said.

Amelia didn't respond, bouncing the car over a speed bump in the hospital parking lot. Everywhere I looked there were police cars. I opened the passenger door before the vehicle was fully stopped. My eyes connected with Bob's as he moved toward me. My feet seemed to defy the command from my mind to move faster. "What happened, Bob?"

He placed both hands on top of my shoulders. In a soothing voice, he explained Gerry was in the examination room with several doctors. "He was on the police bike and responding to a stabbing on the south end of town. An elderly woman pulled out from a parking spot on Martin Street, crossing two lanes of traffic to turn onto a side street. His bike smashed into the side of her car throwing him over the car where he landed head first on the road."

Bob took a deep breath, tipping his head upward in search of some profound answer to my yet unasked questions. There was hurt in his face as his eyebrows pulled tightly together and his large hand covered his eyes.

"His heart stopped..."

I gasped. Bob didn't dare look into my eyes.

My hand covered my mouth. Tenderly, Bob pulled my head to his chest in comfort. "Ssh-Ssh. He's really fighting. He's going to make it. I really believe that and you have to, too. You need to be strong for him," Bob said firmly.

Bob was right. It wouldn't do any good if I fell apart by thinking the worst. Bob scanned the parking lot, taking count of the civilians and police officers lining the sidewalk.

"I'm going to take you to the nurses in Emergency. They're waiting for you. Then I'll go and see what I can find out. Okay?"

Wrapping his arm around my shoulders, Bob guided me inside. I had entered these doors many times looking for a solution to a high fever or sore throat for our children. Gerry had gone in an official capacity many times with prisoners in need of medical attention, or as support for families after an accident, but never, ever, had we entered Emergency grasping only a thread of hope for the survival of our family.

Bob spoke to the nurse, his deep voice echoing over muffled voices in the waiting room. "This is Mrs. Breese. Her husband is the officer who was injured. Do you have a room with some privacy where she can wait?"

Heads turned and eyes, filled with sympathy, offered silent support. "Yes, of course." A woman put down her clipboard and pen and came from behind the counter, sliding her arm around me as Bob moved his away. We walked through the waiting area to a tiny room with a small couch and a square table with a telephone.

"Is there some family that can come to be with you, Mrs. Breese?"

"One of the police officers has gone to get my Mom, and my brother should be arriving soon."

"Fine. Can I get you some coffee, Mrs. Breese? It may be a while before the doctors can see you." I wasn't the least bit concerned with when I could see a doctor - I wanted to see Gerry.

"When...when, can I see my husband?"

The nurse sat down and took my hand in her lap. "A lot of people are working on your husband right now. As soon as they know anything, they'll be in to see you."

She reached behind me for a small box of Kleenex. I pulled some tissue from the box and wiped my nose, and then began to cry uncontrollably.

"Will you be okay for a minute?" the nurse asked with concern.

I was too emotional to answer her and only nodded my head. After the nurse left, I leaned back against the white wall and closed my eyes to avoid the intensity of the fluorescent lighting. My arms and legs ached. I shuddered as a picture of Gerry slamming into the car flashed through my mind. My eyes opened to see several strangers sitting in chairs outside the door, waiting. Did they know what had happened to Gerry and was that why they were looking at me? Or was it because I had made such a scene, crying like a frightened child? Before I could make my mind up to shut the door, the nurse returned with the cup of coffee.

"Here you go. Your family has arrived. They'll be right in."

A hot burning sensation aggravated my already-sour stomach. The oil floating on top of the lukewarm black liquid didn't look appetizing. Seconds later my family came in. The first person I saw was my Mother. Following her were my older sister Rebecca and my sister-in-law Patrice. The last person was Nathan, decked out in his blue uniform. The sudden realization that he was working at the police station when the call came in was too much for me. My throat tightened making it difficult to speak. Warmth and love passed through the room like a surge of electricity as we embraced, letting our pain pour out, as tears from one wet the cheek of the other. The nurse stepped out quietly. Clinging to one another, no words were spoken.

Remembering Brian

We made a list and began notifying relatives and close friends. Each call sent a shock wave through the person receiving the news. At the same time, the caller's fear increased as details of the accident were repeated time and time again. With each call, we promised that we would phone again as soon as we had more information.

The atmosphere was suffused with intense sadness, the same sadness we had endured the year before with the death of my eldest brother, Brian when he was only 39 years old.

Brian and his family lived in Surrey, B.C., six hours away by car. The first time we noticed the obvious deterioration in Brian's health was when he arrived to attend Nathan's RCMP Auxiliary graduation ceremony. We were shocked to see the effects of prescribed medication and quickly understood his decision to travel by bus instead of driving. Brian had been awaiting surgery to correct a work-related injury to his left elbow and a painkiller and anti-depressant had been prescribed to help him through the long wait.

Tragically, the combination of these drugs proved lethal and Brian sustained a subarachnoid hemorrhage. It exploded his brain on both sides, from the inside out, leaving intact only enough of the brain stem to automate his vital organs. He was in a coma with no hope for recovery. The only blessing we could ask for was that he not linger for long in a vegetative state. For me, there was a deep and unnatural pain in wanting him to die, but I knew there was no joy in wanting to keep him alive.

Until now, I had not really understood the magnitude of life changing decisions I had made following his death, or the real reason behind them. In the weeks following this tragedy, I had focused on my own sense of mortality. I kept thinking, "one of us kids" died. Like everyone else, we had prepared ourselves to face the loss of our aging grandparents, and someday our parents...but the thought of one of us kids dying had never occurred to us. This realization rocked me and quickly turned to depression.

I was embarrassed by the intensity of my grief. After all, this loss affected his wife and three children the most. Perhaps, even my mother more so. I was just his little sister. Nonetheless, his death propelled me into making vast changes - changes that frightened even me.

In an attempt to pull myself from this dark hole, it occurred to me that I wanted to spend more time with my husband and children more than anything. I needed to be there for them and, most of all, I didn't want to owe anyone an explanation. These feelings became an obsession as I held close the memory of Brian's devotion to his family. So I began to reshape both my professional and my personal life. First, I took steps to shed the responsibilities of my volunteer work in the community. Then I quit my job with an accounting firm and made plans to open a bookkeeping business from home. With each change, I felt more in control of my destiny.

There was one problem. I wasn't prepared for my family's reaction. Foremost was Gerry's decided unhappiness that I had quit my job. However, he began to feel at ease after seeing my quick accumulation of bookkeeping clients. My monthly income doubled in less than five months, but the ultimate pay-off was that I was now fully accessible to Gerry and our daughters. At any given time I could be there if they needed me. No questions asked. All I needed to do was work my clients around my schedule.

Tonight, the importance of being available to my family became even clearer as we waited for the doctors to give us a report on Gerry's injuries. Brian's death 14 months earlier had brought about changes in my life which would significantly benefit Gerry in his recovery. All the changes had been for a reason – a very definite reason.

The door suddenly opened.

"Hello, Mrs. Breese? I'm Dr. Wright. I would like to speak with you about your husband before you see him."

I clutched his hand, anxious to hear what he had to say, yet not wanting to be separated from Gerry for another minute. "Hi. Please call me Janelle. This is my family," I said introducing each by name. Dr. Wright pointed towards the sofa. "Please have a seat, Mrs. Breese."

"How is my husband, Dr. Wright? Have you been able to stabilize him?"

Dr. Wright lifted his hand, gently instructing me to slow down.

"First things first. Let me explain what's happened. Are you aware your husband's heart stopped at the accident scene?"

"Yes, I was told two bystanders administered CPR."

"That's correct." Dr. Wright lowered his eyes and eyebrows as he studied the back of one hand. "Both of them are trained paramedics. We are certain his heart has been stabilized."

"That's good, right?" I was elated.

Dr. Wright straightened in his chair and adjusted his watchband. "It is good. But he's not out of the woods yet." Looking into my eyes, he warned, "Your husband is in critical condition, Mrs. Breese, with very serious injuries - the most serious being a brain injury. He has a contusion on the frontal lobes, which is like a big bruise. The severe shaking of his brain against his skull when he hit the pavement caused the bruising. He needs to have a CT Scan done to determine how much swelling there is in the brain. Unfortunately, we don't have a Scanner in Penticton so he needs to be transported to Kelowna."

"Will he come back to Penticton after the test is done?" I asked.

"No. Dr. Huang is a specialist in Kelowna, an expert in this area. I've spoken to him and he's prepared to assume the care for your husband."

"How long will he be there?"

Dr. Wright stretched his hands out to clamp his palms onto his knees. "That depends on your husband. Each brain injury is different and the timing varies dramatically. As long as he remains in a coma, he will remain in Kelowna. As soon as he is awake and stable, he will be transferred back to Penticton."

My mother looked very concerned. I could tell she feared the worst.

"How long will Gerry be in the hospital when he gets back to Penticton?"

"Again, that depends on your husband, Mrs. Breese. What your brain will do is different than what my brain would do, given the exact same injury. We'll just have to wait and see."

Those three final words grated on my nerves bringing to mind my conversations with Ruth and her frustrations in being told to "wait and see." Determined to be the one in control, I pressed Dr. Wright for more information.

"What is happening with him right now? Can I see him?"

"You can — in time. At the moment we are attempting to get x-rays so we can rule out any internal bleeding and spinal injuries. He is struggling and fighting, so it's very difficult to work with him."

"Fighting?! Isn't he in a coma?"

Dr Wright leaned back. "He is in a coma. But he is also in tremendous pain and that's why he's fighting. We suspect he has multiple broken bones and possibly a broken jaw. It appears all his teeth are broken. He'll require dental surgery."

I cringed. He continued, looking at me intensely. "Your husband skidded on his face across the pavement so he has extensive facial lacerations which require plastic surgery. I have explained this to Dr. Huang. He will be contacting Dr. Knight, a plastic surgeon. We expect to be transporting your husband by ambulance within the next two hours. You should make arrangements for yourself. I'll notify the hospital in Kelowna that you'll be arriving tonight." Dr. Wright excused himself, promising someone would take me to Intensive Care to see Gerry soon.

There was so much to do. First of all, I had to make arrangements for the girls to be taken care of and to notify my bookkeeping clients that I would be unavailable for at least a week. My sister, Rebecca retrieved paper and pen to make a list.

The heavy thud of boots sounded outside the doorway. It was Bob Ogden and a nurse.

"Hello, Mrs. Breese. Corporal Ogden and I will take you to your husband now. He is in ICU, so I can only allow you and one other person to go up."

Another nurse waited just inside the doorway to prepare me for what I was going to see. Her voice was low and steady. "Be prepared to see four men holding your husband. Two are medical staff and two are police officers. Try not to let this upset you. We're going to give him some medication to try to calm him down but, unfortunately, we're unable to give him any painkillers right now. He needs to see the doctor in Kelowna first and have the CT Scan done. He's got very bad facial injuries as well so he is not very pleasant to look at right now." She paused briefly before continuing. "His nose is broken. He has extremely deep gashes around the mouth area. The deepest laceration is to his chin which has left a gaping hole beneath his lower lip."

I felt sick. It was impossible to imagine how Gerry looked. Trying to maintain my composure, I shifted from one foot to the other, briefly nodding to an orderly as he walked past. The nurse didn't acknowledge the passerby. Instead she kept her eyes on me and continued to explain Gerry's injuries. "Also, we have a cervical collar on him. That will remain in place until we ascertain if he has a spinal injury or not." She hesitated. "Are you okay, Mrs. Breese? Do you think you can go in and face this?"

"I'm okay," I assured her. "I really need to see him."

I was lying and I knew it. There was no doubt I needed, and wanted, to see him but, in reality, I wasn't ready to see his devastating injuries. We walked down the corridor by the nurses' station. As we approached the curtained room I could hear Gerry moaning. He sounded frightened and it scared me. When we reached the doorway, the nurse pulled back the curtains giving me full view of the room and the people inside.

Gerry was lying on a stretcher with the top slightly raised. His shirt had been ripped open and electrodes were stuck on his chest. His boots and socks had been removed. Two police officers stood on his left side and two medical personnel stood on the right, holding him down just as the nurse had said. There were several nurses and our family doctor in the small room as well. Everyone was watching and waiting for my reaction. Suddenly, I wasn't as calm as I thought.

I was familiar with only one officer, Randy Kirkoski. My eyes met his, but I was unable to speak. The officer whom I hadn't met was Corporal Cy Kelly. I moved closer to the stretcher and stood between the officers. This was my first clear view of Gerry's facial injuries. Blood oozed from his gaping chin. His nose was bloodied and already swollen from the break. His puffy eyes were shut. Trembling, I reached to stroke his hair. My chest felt tight. I was shocked to see how battered he was.

My fingers caressed his hair. I was embarrassed as everyone watched me lean forward to whisper in his ear. I wanted to hold him, caress him, and tell him I loved him. His moans made me anxious and I wanted to do anything to stop his pain. When I first said his name he didn't hear me. I spoke louder not caring who heard me this time.

"Gerry, it's me, Janelle. I'm right here, Honey. Everything's going to be okay."

Hearing my words, Gerry bolted upward letting out a tremendous scream. He tried to pull his arms away from the men. It was frightening to watch. I jumped and started to cry, pulling my hand away as if I were responsible. Officer Kelly maintained a firm grip on Gerry's leg while two other men tried to force him back down. Cy leaned over, his head touching mine, offering words of encouragement.

"It's okay. He knows it's you. Just keep talking to him."

I looked at Cy, again feeling embarrassed. I had let this upset me. It hadn't occurred to me that he had screamed because he recognized my voice. Again I touched his head. My throat tightened. No words came. Suddenly, without warning the room began to tilt and my vision blurred. A hot flash rushed through my body. My balance was unsteady. Dr. Quandt stepped forward taking my arm to guide me to a chair. He told me to put my head between my knees and breathe slowly. I wanted to vomit. My dignity ebbed away as I breathed deeply, fanning myself for some air.

Bob Ogden helped me from the chair and suggested he take me back to sit with my family. Mom and Rebecca were waiting for us at the end of the darkened hallway outside the intensive care unit. He patiently answered their questions about Gerry before encouraging them to take me downstairs into the waiting room. Memories raced through my mind, flickering like a candle flame caught in a draft. Each one struggled to keep alive and burn brightly, regardless of the odds.

Gerry's younger brother, the only surviving member of his immediate family had arrived. Dan, three years younger than me, was born with mild cerebral palsy and has slight physical and emotional difficulties. My mother quickly stepped in upon his arrival, answering his questions. She tried to ease his fears and yet wanted to be honest about the seriousness of his brother's medical condition.

The nurse from ICU came downstairs to see us. She smiled warmly resting a hand on my shoulder. "Mrs. Breese, the ambulance to transport your husband to Kelowna has arrived. We'll be bringing him through momentarily."

"Could my family and his brother see him before he leaves?" I asked.

"Well, briefly. There isn't a tremendous amount of time, so when he comes through Emergency just ask the attendants to stop for a minute. But please, keep it brief."

The elevator bell sounded and the doors opened. Two ambulance attendants maneuvered a gurney through the steel doorway frame. Nurses followed. One walked alongside holding a bag of intravenous liquid. Gerry was completely still, almost lifeless. They wheeled him closer. Not a sound. No moaning, no struggle. Fear gripped me.

"He's not making a sound anymore. What's happened?" I said tugging on the nurse's arm.

"Oh … I'm sorry. I should have explained that you would see a difference in him from upstairs. We weren't able to give him painkillers because the neurologist in Kelowna needs to see him first, so we gave him some Valium to sedate him."

The attendants hurried past us, not stopping as promised. Their determination to reach their destination showed. Interrupting them seemed inappropriate. Instead, my family and I followed outside and gathered around the open doors of the ambulance while they loaded Gerry into the back. A look of horror crept over each one's face as their eyes fell upon his bruised and bloodied body.

Dan began to shiver and weave. A nurse rushed toward him with a wheelchair. My body froze, preventing me from going to him or showing any sign of compassion or understanding. The nurse patted Dan's hand and knelt down beside the wheelchair to explain Gerry's injuries. I turned to ask the attendant if I could go inside the ambulance to speak to Gerry before they left. He said yes, but I'd have to be brief.

I climbed into the back and hunched over the stretcher. Gerry's eyes were closed, his face expressionless. My love for him poured out as my trembling hand gently caressed his black and blue cheek.

"I love you, Gerry. Please don't be frightened. I can't travel in the ambulance with you because I need to go see Myriah and Dale. They don't know what has happened yet. I want to be the one to explain it to them. As soon as I get them settled with Bob and Ruth, I'll come to Kelowna." My eyes burned. He lay still on the stretcher not making a sound, nor responding to my touch. "I love you. I'll be with you all the way."

Gently, I kissed him on the forehead. As I lifted my head, bright red blood started to gush from his nose. It startled me. The attendant beside me quickly moved in, using a cloth to soak it up.

"Sorry. You'll have to step outside now. We have to go," the attendant stated abruptly. The attendant outside the ambulance reached for my arm to help me down. As my feet hit the pavement the same attendant brushed past me, climbing inside the ambulance quickly, making the transfer of our bodies appear seamless. The driver slammed both doors shut and jumped in the front seat. Within seconds, the lights on the top of the vehicle began to turn, streaking the night sky with wisps of glowing red. The wheels made a crunching sound as the treads flattened loose dirt and gravel into the pavement.

I stood with my family and friends watching my husband being carried away. As the red flashing lights became fainter in the distance, I wondered if their disappearance into the cold black night was symbolic of the disappearance of the strong able bodied man I loved.

Wait and See

It was nearly 2:00 a.m. before we arrived at Kelowna General Hospital. Corporal Sanderson, the traffic analyst, drove the cruiser in silence. Mom sat hushed in the back seat separated from us by the plexiglass used to prevent contact with prisoners. While I was cognizant of the Corporal beside me, I made no effort to talk. At the main entrance, Corporal Sanderson retrieved our luggage from the trunk. He wished us well and handed me his business card, assuring me that I should call if I needed anything. I thanked him and promised to keep everyone informed of Gerry's progress.

Inside the lobby we asked for directions to the Intensive Care Unit. A security officer, clad in gray-blue uniform, offered to escort us. I felt conscious of people staring and wondered if they were wondering why we were going to the dreaded ICU. My feet shuffled into the elevator. Daylight was only a few hours away. I was exhausted but had no desire to sleep. All I wanted was to be near my husband to give him all the strength I could. The guard pointed to an intercom panel on the wall outside the double doors that led to the ICU. "Ring the buzzer to have a nurse let you in."

There was no sound when I pushed the button, but within seconds a voice came over the speaker. I spoke my name into the silver box and explained I was there to sit with my husband. The voice replied, confused. I explained again who I was. Quite unexpectedly, a loud sigh returned over the speaker and the female voice said she would be right out.

"Mrs.Breese?"

I nodded and introduced my mother, feeling relieved she now understood who we were.

"Do you have a place to stay?" The tone in her voice was more than just concern. Perhaps our late night arrival was just one more thing to do.

"No, not yet." I tried not to sound defensive. "We'll look for a motel in the morning, but I want to be sure of my husband's condition before leaving him alone."

The nurse replied firmly, "That's fine for tonight. We do have some foam mats that you may use if you like. However, we strongly encourage families to find suitable accommodations once the initial danger has passed, usually by the second day."

My defenses went up, my frayed nerves toughened. She was in control of the rules here, but it was *my husband* lying beyond those doors. Before she could challenge me any further, I inquired about how he did in the ambulance and asked if the specialist had seen him. I picked up my suitcase and stepped closer to the doors, waiting for her to answer. The nurse paused. Briefly, we stood toe to toe before she stepped aside and let us enter.

Beyond the doors a long, dark hallway with a glossy tiled floor stretched before us. At the end of it, dim lights hovered over a nurse writing at a desk. I could barely make out two beds with elderly women hooked up to machines and intravenous poles. I anxiously peered into doorways looking for Gerry as we followed the nurse down the hallway. As we walked she explained that the neurosurgeon would be by in the morning. He had been notified of Gerry's arrival at Kelowna General, but did not feel it was necessary to come and examine him at this late hour.

Did this mean Gerry was no longer listed in serious condition? No. He was in serious but stable condition. If there were any change, the specialist would indeed come sooner. I was relieved to hear that.

She guided me to the bed where Gerry lay on his back with pillows tucked beneath his left side. I stopped and stared. The sheet covering him was folded at the waist, leaving his chest exposed. He was connected to a heart monitor. A tiny computerized heart flashed on the screen. How I loved him! I smiled at the tiny heart as it winked in a slow steady rhythm. Its dance was the dance of life and its silent song filled my heart. The nurse smiled as I wiped away my tears. She explained that propping him up with pillows helped him breathe. There was a definite change in the tone of her voice, now sympathetic and warm.

Besides the heart monitor, he had an airway inserted in his mouth and an intravenous tube in his left arm. The airway, covered by an oxygen mask, looked odd. Why did he need oxygen when he was breathing through an airway? The nurse told me the mask was needed to keep the loose bandages on his chin moist until the plastic surgery could be done.

Gerry seemed much more peaceful. I noticed his right hand was tremendously swollen. When I asked the nurse if it was broken, she seemed surprised at the puffiness and promised to note it on his chart for the doctor to assess in the morning. I was puzzled why the staff hadn't noticed the obvious swelling.

While gently stroking his hair, I scanned his body in search of other injuries. There were massive scratches running across his chest and stomach. A large cut on his left elbow was also covered with a loose bandage. His skin felt warm, seemingly unchanged by the chill I felt in the air. The dim lights cast shadows over the bed, but I could clearly see the extensive bruising was beginning to create large splashes of color all over his body. I leaned over the cold metal railing to tenderly kiss his forehead. There was no response as I grazed his ear and whispered his name.

"Is he in a coma?"

"Yes, he is."

Gerry was classified as a 5 on the Glasgow Coma Scale, a measurement used to determine the intensity of a coma. The most severe brain injury is three to eight on the scale, a moderate brain injury nine to twelve, and a minor brain injury, thirteen to fifteen. The measurements are based on a combination of verbal and motor responses. Some of the factors considered are: eye opening, motor or physical movement, and verbal responses.

"How long will he be in a coma?"

"Each brain injury is different," she said. "We'll just have to wait and see."

I had already heard this term "Wait and see," and I had a definite feeling it would become a constant echo in the days ahead. Sighing, I pulled a chair to his bedside. The nurse took Mom to show her where the foam mats were. It was the first time since the accident that Gerry and I were left alone. It was quiet and comforting in a strange way -

comforting to sit and think about our lives, comforting to pray in complete solitude, comforting to know he was alive.

Mom returned with a different nurse. The chaplain for the RCMP was waiting in the hallway to see me. I was surprised. In all our years with the police, I had no idea there was a local chaplain. Most of all, I was astonished he had heard of our situation so soon.

"This is the ICU ward and people outside the immediate family are not permitted," she explained sharply, walking down the hallway in front of me. "I've told him this, but he wants to speak to you. Please arrange to have one person for your contact. Your husband's only been here a short time and already we've had several phone calls. It's not so much a problem at the moment, but the nursing staff during the day will simply not have the time."

My cheeks flushed with embarrassment. I was not a child to be reprimanded. Of course I knew these people were busy. It was beyond my control that someone had come to see me. The chaplain was just doing his job by offering support to families and members of the police force. How I didn't want to be continually defending myself!

A tall lean man waited at the end of the corridor. His name was Tim Schroeder and I liked him immediately. Tim had learned of us from the Kelowna RCMP, and he offered to do anything he could to help. He asked that I keep him informed of Gerry's progress and hoped they would meet each other one day. At the time I thought this conversation would probably be the extent of our relationship. Little did I know, but Tim would come back into our lives sooner rather than later.

Mom went downstairs to have a cigarette after Tim left. I went back into the ICU ward to be at Gerry's side.

"I'll say one thing for sure," the same nurse said as I approached Gerry's bed where she was checking his intravenous line, "The police force certainly do take care of their own."

I nodded, giving her a frail smile. "It's sort of an unwritten law. When a police officer's family needs help, everyone pitches in."

She smiled, tapping her fingers on the bed-rails and then spun on her heels. "Yeah, it's nice!"

It was now the wee hours of the morning. Mom and I stood on either side of the bed. Gerry made no sound nor did he move. The nurse at the desk suggested we go and lie down for a while. It sounded good. Even if I couldn't sleep it would feel good just to rest my legs and back. Mom agreed.

"Gerry, it's four thirty in the morning. You've been in an accident and we're at the hospital. I'm really tired. Mom and I are going into the next room to lie down. I'll be back soon." Leaving a gentle peck on his cheek, I turned to walk away.

Suddenly, Gerry moaned and thrashed his arms. The computerized heart flashed, the monitor beeped, alerting the medical personnel. His nurse rushed from her desk and pressed quickly down on the electrodes attached to his chest while keeping a constant eye on the monitor. My eyes studied her face for any sign of what might be happening. Adrenaline pumped through my body and I panicked thinking he was in jeopardy once more.

"Sometimes when he moves quickly it loosens the patches," she said, addressing my unspoken fear. The machine kept beeping. The nurse slowly checked each patch. Her comments relieved me. I moved closer to the bed taking Gerry's hand in mine.

"It's okay, Honey. I'm right here. It's okay." His moans quieted and the flashing heart slowed down. The beeps finally stopped when Gerry's heartbeat settled at a normal rate.

The nurse smiled. "See, he knows you're here. He knew that was your touch."

I was amazed. How could he tell? Did he understand what I was saying when I told him we were going to lie down for a while? Was he showing me he wanted me to stay? We stayed at his side for another 45 minutes. This time, when I decided to leave, I simply motioned for Mom to follow me.

Two hours later, we were up and waiting for the doctors to make their morning rounds. It was tedious pacing back and forth alongside Gerry's bed. Each time someone new entered the unit my hopes rose. And those hopes were quickly shattered each time it was someone else's doctor. My requests for information had already caused the nurses to give short blunt answers, usually ending in the wearisome "wait and see." I was annoyed and frustrated. Surely I wasn't the first family member to ask for explicit information.

At no time did I profess to have expert knowledge about the medical procedures used in treating brain injuries. But I wanted, and needed, to learn. I have never taken small engine mechanics but I wouldn't dream of letting a mechanic perform major repairs on my vehicle without first hearing an explanation of why it must be done. Furthermore, if I didn't understand the explanation I wouldn't hesitate to ask for clarification. I had to hold onto the faith that I was an intelligent person. As my questions kept coming, I didn't intend them as insults to the competency of the medical people. Rather, I needed answers to get through what was happening.

Finally Dr. Knight, the plastic surgeon, arrived - a small gray-haired man with soft eyes, readily revealing a gentle nature. His compassion was confirmed as he examined Gerry and carefully manipulated the bandages. Dr. Knight worked quickly and then took the time to explain what he was planning to do.

"Your husband needs surgery to close those cuts. At the same time, I'll correct his broken nose. I don't believe his jaw is broken, but I'll know for certain after we take x-rays. The ones taken the night of the accident didn't show all we need and, apparently, he was too agitated to obtain more. The nurses noted on his chart that you're concerned his right hand is broken. From looking at it, I think you might be right so I'll have my colleague, an orthopedic surgeon, attend during the surgery. It will be easier to set and cast it while he's under anesthetic."

"Could the surgery wait for a while, Dr. Knight, until he is out of a coma?" I asked. As long as I had known him, Gerry hadn't undergone surgery.

"Well, the gash on his elbow definitely requires stitching. The upper lip is split in half and the chin area below his lower lip is cut through to the bottom layer crosswise which also requires extensive repair. Considering the severity of those cuts, I really believe your husband is at a far greater risk from complications due to infection than he is from undergoing an anesthetic."

A Change of Mind

"Okay." I tried to put my mind at ease. "I'm concerned about his foot too," I added, walking to the foot of the bed and lifting the once crisp, white sheet that was now splattered with blood. The left foot looked quite black.

Dr. Knight grimaced at the sight. From his expression, I assumed either the nursing staff had not indicated the condition of Gerry's foot on the chart or, Dr. Knight had overlooked any comments on it. "My goodness, it really is black and blue, isn't it?" The bruising appeared darkest from the ankle down the front to the toes and lightest on the sole of his foot. From a side view, the gradual changes in color gave the bruising a layered effect. Gerry moaned, trying to pull his foot away.

"I'm sorry, Gerry. I know it must be quite sore," the doctor said. "I don't know if it's broken Mrs. Breese, but he definitely has massive bruises. I think it would be best to have it x-rayed at the same time they x-ray his face and hand. Then we'll know for sure. Just be prepared though – as time goes along, you'll probably notice more and more bruises. Sometimes, bruising can be so severe that it takes longer to heal than a broken bone."

"Really?" I asked in disbelief. "It never occurred to me that bruising could be worse than a break."

"Well, it can be and I suspect that is what has happened with your husband."

Footsteps approached the bed. It was one of the nurses and a doctor. The nurse introduced him as Dr. Huang, the neurosurgeon.

"Mrs. Breese? Your husband?" he asked looking at me first, then pointing towards Gerry.

"What do you think?" Dr. Huang asked Dr. Knight.

The plastic surgeon explained his plans for surgery, along with his reasons for not wanting to wait until the coma had lifted. Dr. Huang listened, moving his head up and down, saying: "Yeah, Yeah, Yeah."

Dr. Knight stepped aside. Dr. Huang placed a hand on Gerry's chest, rubbing vigorously. "Gerry! You are in the hospital. You have been in a bad accident on your police bike. You have a brain injury."

Gerry moaned and swung his right leg to kick the doctor. Dr. Huang pushed the leg down and then opened Gerry's eyes, shining a small flashlight to see how reactive his pupils were. "Gerry, you have been in bad accident. On your motorcycle." Dr. Huang released Gerry's eyelids, tucked the small flashlight back into his pocket and rubbed his fist on Gerry's chest even more aggressively. Gerry thrashed his legs.

I felt so protective. I knew the doctor was testing his responses and the depth of the coma, but I didn't like seeing Gerry so aggravated. "It's okay, Gerry. I'm right here. Dr. Huang needs to examine you. He's going to take care of you." I felt I was intruding on the doctor's territory. Dr. Huang simply watched and then shook Gerry's shoulder. Gerry was a big man and trained to fight back. He kicked and swung his leg hard, this time connecting with the nurse at the foot of the bed. Teetering, she grasped the foot rail. This behavior was so unlike the gentle natured man I married. The nurse and doctors made no comment so I didn't know if this was typical behavior with a brain injury or if Gerry was simply being uncooperative. My eyes were burning from tears. Taking his hand, I whispered into his ear, "It's okay, Honey. Dr. Huang needs to examine you so he can help you."

Without any further struggle Gerry lowered his leg and rested his hand in mine, making only a low soft moaning sound as I stroked his fingers. My eyes connected with Dr. Huang. Instead of asking me to leave the room as I thought he would, Dr. Huang smiled. "My goodness, he knows it's you. Yes, he knows. He can tell difference between you and me," the doctor encouraged.

Dr. Huang's comments made me immensely happy and relieved. I wiped away a tear, exhaustion sweeping my body. Silently I waited for Dr. Huang to offer an assessment. When it became apparent he wasn't going to, I asked how long he felt the coma would last and what, if any, the permanent deficits would be. His reply was like all the others.

"Well, you understand ... each brain injury is different. What his brain does is different than someone else's. I can't tell you how long. We just have to wait and see."

Wait and see! WAIT AND SEE! WA-A-IT AND SE-E-E-!!! I wanted to scream. Why couldn't anyone say something concrete?

A Change of Mind

Something I could understand – something I could hold on to. I desperately wanted just one solid piece of information to grasp onto, so I'd know what was going to happen. The frustration was unbearable. If he had broken bones or needed his gallbladder removed doctors could comment on the estimated length of recovery, but with a brain injury the best anyone could say is, "We'll just have to wait and see!"

"Please, Dr. Huang. Can you at least tell me why sometimes he thrashes his arms and legs and other times he doesn't move a muscle?"

Now even Dr. Huang stiffened in reaction to my pressure. "He in a deep coma now. Sometimes a coma lightens and then it deepens. This is normal," was his reply. Before I could continue, he picked up the chart from the foot of the bed and walked away. I burst into tears, turning to seek comfort from my mother.

"Normal! None of this is normal! I just want to know what's going to happen to us?"

A nurse came over and urged us to leave. But I felt I had to spend every minute with Gerry. What if he came out of the coma and I wasn't there? What if he took a turn for the worse and I wasn't there? The nurse wouldn't take no for an answer, explaining that taking a break, even for a few minutes at a time, was essential to my own well-being. I agreed, reluctantly. However, I wanted to spend just a few minutes alone with him before I left. The nurse and my mother made me promise that I would stay no more than two minutes.

Standing alone beside his bed, the tears streamed down my face. How could this be? My husband was rugged, full of life, enjoyed the outdoors, drank beer with his buddies, cuddled his children, and was very proud of his position as a police officer. He was my best friend and lover. The man lying before me was unable to even communicate.

It was true – all we could do was wait and see.

A Change of Mind

The Touching Sound
of Hello

The white enamel doors of the Intensive Care Unit felt heavy as my weary arms pushed them open. My body ached from exhaustion, as did my mind, saturated with thoughts and concerns for our family and our future. Most of the thoughts surfaced out of my own fears. I couldn't seem to shake the fear because I lacked any information on brain injuries and what I should or shouldn't expect. It felt incredibly lonely and scary.

Stepping out of the ICU into the hospital corridor, I was startled by the sound of a deep yet familiar voice.

"Hi there, gorgeous!"

It was Bob MacMillan, a Penticton fireman, and our neighbor. Standing beside him was Gerry's Staff Sargent, Jack MacDonald and his wife Mary. My eyes widened, then filled with tears at the thought of them traveling sixty kilometers to Kelowna just to see me - especially when they knew they wouldn't be allowed to visit Gerry.

We clung to one another and I struggled to answer their many questions. Ironically, in trying to sound neither too morbid nor overly optimistic, I found myself using the phrase I despised. "Wait and see" sent a shiver down my back as it came out of my mouth. Surely they would want to know something more. I waited for them to press me for more details. They didn't. Instead they seemed quite satisfied with the small amount of information I was able to give.

The elevator bell rang. We stopped talking and mindlessly watched people exit the elevator. To my surprise and delight, two more familiar faces came into view. It was my brother Nathan and his wife Patrice and with them were a man and woman I had yet to meet. My brother introduced the man as an RCMP Inspector stationed here in Kelowna and his wife. He had come to pay the respects of his detachment and to offer any assistance that we might need. His wife handed me their home phone number, encouraging me to call day or night for any reason at all. The conversation with our new acquaintances was brief but very warming. Words can't explain how comforting it was to see so many familiar faces, as well as having the caring thoughts of people I had never met.

Immediately after the Inspector and his wife departed, Nathan insisted we go for lunch and then check into the motel where we had reservations. The thought of food repulsed me, but I didn't stand a chance of not going with him.

"Come on Janelle. You've got to eat and you need a break. It isn't going to do Gerry any good if you wear yourself out." His eyes twinkled. No matter how discouraging life seemed, I couldn't resist his smile. "Besides," he continued, "I'm not going to take no for an answer!"

"I can see that," I said, laughing for the first time.

One of the nurses had been listening to Nathan's efforts to persuade me to leave. She tapped me on the shoulder, reminding me that I had already given them the motel's phone number so they could call if there was any change. She even suggested a nearby restaurant. Together, Nathan and the nurse made it very difficult for me to resist. During lunch, I emptied my coffee cup several times and did little more than push my salad around the plate. My family kept the conversation light, but my mind centered on thoughts of Gerry alone in the hospital.

I was relieved when Nathan suggested we go to the motel. The sooner we checked in, the sooner we could go back to the hospital. The motel owners, informed of our situation, greeted us with sympathy and compassion. To my surprise, the desk clerk handed me nearly a dozen phone messages. I thought only a few people knew where we were staying and most of them were with me. The wife escorted us to our room. It was like an apartment, boasting a living room with two hide-a-beds, a dining area and a kitchen complete with dishwasher and microwave, a bathroom, and a bedroom with a queen size bed. Nathan offered to make coffee while I freshened up.

Without even looking into the mirror, I sensed this overnight ordeal had aged me well beyond my 34 years. I turned on the taps, letting the warm water trickle across my fingers. It felt so good. I cupped it in my hands and splashed my face. As I patted the hand towel on my skin, I heard new voices coming from the other room.

When I opened the door to peek around the corner, I couldn't believe my eyes. Gerry's entire shift had arrived! They had decided to bring up my car, making it easier for us to get to and from the hospital, day or night. It was a great idea. Up to that point, I hadn't even considered what we would do about transportation. I made my way across the room, giving each a hug and a kiss. Gerry would be so proud to know Bob Ogden had come, along with Amelia Hayden, Hughie Winters, and a fellow I'd not met before. Bob introduced him as Bryce Peterson.

Nathan passed around cups of coffee to everyone while Hughie explained the hospital staff had given them the address. The conversation quickly turned to Gerry. Each one asked questions, only some of which I could answer. Working through their shock, one by one they explained where they were and what they were doing when the call came in about the accident. It was easy to sense their tremendous bond as a team. Unlike any other group Gerry had worked with in his career as a police officer, these people really cared about one another and they truly loved working together. I took a moment to silently enjoy the relationship Gerry had with each of them.

First there was Bob Ogden, the shift supervisor. He and Ruth were our closest friends. We harbored a deep respect for Bob, which came from watching him nurture Ruth back to health after her accident, never faltering in his love. Gerry also held Bob in high esteem for being an excellent street cop.

Next was Amelia. She had the unpleasant task of notifying me about Gerry's accident. Still considered a rookie, Amelia had been dealt her fair share of office pranks with Gerry often the one responsible. Nevertheless, Amelia admired Gerry and often sought his brotherly advice about work or her personal life. Gerry had equal respect for Amelia. He praised her for taking her job so seriously, carrying a full load of responsibilities. To him, she was one of the guys. He was flattered when she asked him for advice, especially when she used it.

Bryce had recently moved to Penticton and had not experienced the full range of fun and games that this group was capable of. However, his compassion was visible as he offered prayers for the full recovery of his new coworker and friend.

Hughie was probably the closest to Gerry. They were partners on the job and partners in the pranks too! They were always laughing, always scheming. But putting aside all the fun and games, there wasn't any doubt when they were working. They could count on each other. In testimony to his keen sense of humor, Hughie lightened the atmosphere by making a list of errands.

"We're at your disposal, Janelle. Let us take over the mundane details."

It was difficult to organize my thoughts. "Gosh, Hugh. I don't know where to begin," I stumbled. The dark haired mischievous jester leaned back in the chair, stretching his hands behind his head. "How about underwear?" We all started to laugh. "Tell me which drawer you keep them in and I'll be happy to see that all your sexiest lingerie is brought here," he continued while managing to keep a straight face.

"Thanks, you are very kind," I assured him. "But I think I'll make out just fine with what I packed," I replied, remembering how hectic it was the night before packing for myself and the girls.

Getting down to serious business, I suggested he contact a lawyer. The lawyer we had for the past ten years was no longer in practice. Hugh didn't think it was something I should be concerned with at the moment. However, I persisted.

"You know what insurance companies are like, Hugh. Sooner or later someone will approach me and I'd just as soon have a lawyer to direct those calls to. Call someone and ask if they will act on my behalf. I'll personally contact them when we return home." Hugh glanced around the room. "How about Gordie Marshall, Bob? Gerry thinks a lot of him in court," he asked.

Bob, leaning against the wall with arms folded across his chest, replied, "Yeah, Gordie's a good guy. Gerry gets along with him."

Not another word was said. For the time being, all the frustration I'd harbored the past twenty-four hours seemed to drift away. These are true friends, I thought.

This lull didn't last long. The next few days proved to be a true test. The frustration mounted as we waited for signs of Gerry's coma to lift.

A Change of Mind

He had begun to run a low grade fever, indicating that Dr. Knight's fear of an infection setting in had indeed become a reality. It was necessary to move up scheduling his plastic surgery to prevent further complications.

I sat holding his hand, reflecting on our life together, waiting for the nurses to take him downstairs to surgery. He had been through so much in his thirty-seven years. Both his parents died before his 21st birthday. In 1979, two days after learning I was pregnant with our second child, Gerry's younger brother Dale was viciously murdered by a guy he had chummed with for years. This was more pain than anyone should endure. Fortunately though, we had lots of happy memories, too.

We met July 2, 1974, in Surrey, B.C. This large municipality located on the outskirts of Vancouver, B.C., was Gerry's first posting. Gerry was twenty years old and finished his police training only two weeks earlier. Upon his arrival in town, he randomly selected the motel where my family and I were staying while waiting to move into our new house. At seventeen years old, I thought I knew what love was. But it wasn't until I met him that I felt it.

Two years later, we married. Typical newlyweds, we didn't have much money. A rookie's pay was about $750.00 per month and I worked as a bank teller, earning less than five hundred dollars a month. It didn't matter. We were happy and our lives were filled with laughter and dreams.

In our free time, we took leisurely walks along the beach or spent hours driving around looking at dream homes. Whenever Gerry had weekends off, we got together with my parents, brothers and sisters and their spouses. The men would gather in the family room for a session of fifty cent poker and the women visited around the kitchen table.

I loved him. Our children loved him. For the first time, I wasn't thanking God that we had met. Instead I was challenging Him, asking what we had done to deserve being plunged into this dark hole. My hand glided over Gerry's arm, sensitive to the warmth of his skin. There was so much to tell him. Suddenly I felt as though I hadn't told him enough how much I loved him or how proud I was to be his wife. But try as I might, the words wouldn't come. Instead I lowered the rail to lean forward and rest my head on his chest until I felt a gentle tap on my shoulder. It was Gerry's nurse.

"Mrs. Breese, they're coming upstairs for your husband now. We have a few things to do. Perhaps you could say your goodbyes and then wait outside."

Her words stung! "… say your good-byes…" be damned, I thought. For three days I had been holding death's door shut with all my might, begging God to not let Gerry slip through and here she was telling me to say my goodbyes. It made walking away from his bed at that moment the hardest thing I had ever done.

The two hour surgery seemed like an eternity. I paced up and down the hallway. The nurses and Mom finally convinced me to go downstairs to the cafeteria for coffee and a sandwich. It was all I could do to stay down there for the short time that we did. We had just returned when an orderly wheeled Gerry from the elevator, Dr. Knight just steps behind them. I tried to catch a glimpse of Gerry while the man pushed the stretcher through the ICU doors.

"He did fine, just fine." Dr. Knight's gentle words soothed me. He asked us to be seated in the waiting room so he could explain everything that was done.

"You'll see he has a plaster cast on his nose as well as one on his right hand. His nose was broken but the hand wasn't. It was the base of the thumb that was shattered. It should heal without any trouble." Dr. Knight leaned back in his chair, taking a moment to review his thoughts before continuing. Slowly, I tapped my foot, trying to suppress the urge to tell him to "go on." He took a pen from his jacket and reached for some tissue nearby. With that he constructed a sketch of the surgery.

"He required stitches on the inside and the outside of his upper lip, under his bottom lip, down the center of his chin and his elbow. We found the cuts on his left arm and left leg weren't deep enough to stitch so I put butterfly tapes on them. I took a good look inside his mouth and, surprising enough, not a tooth was missing nor was his jaw broken."

Amazingly, none of his teeth were broken. What a relief that was. Before leaving, Dr. Knight asked to see Gerry in about eight weeks for a check-up. His comments led me to believe he felt Gerry would be out of the coma and back home by then.

Gerry's personal nurse, Gail, was waiting at the doorway when I returned. She smiled. "You should see a big difference now."

She was right. I did. The difference in part was my attitude. Things didn't seem so bad now that the surgery was over. I walked softly to the top of his bed hoping not to disturb him. He made no sound, never moved. His swollen eyelids were a vivid purple and yellow. The large white plaster cast on his nose made him look like a hockey goalie. His face was quite swollen where it was stitched; but it looked much better compared to the gaping wounds before surgery,

We waited late into the night for some change. Only the next morning did Gerry show signs of improvement. Immediately, I noticed he readily responded to my voice and touch. The changes were restricted to me, however. He kicked at the nurses when they tried to suction his airway and by late afternoon he seemed to be agitated with the catheter and the intravenous line. Finally the staff applied arm restraints to protect him from further injury. I wondered if Gerry's reactions indicated he was waking from the coma. Dr. Huang wouldn't commit himself when I asked, but he did say it was a very good sign.

That night, I asked the nurse if I could give him a sponge bath. She was delighted, suggesting he probably would prefer it, considering how he instinctively knew the difference between our touches.

I pulled the curtain closed around his bed and lifted back the white sheet. Dr. Knight had warned me there would be more bruises as time went by. How right he was! Gerry's entire body was streaked with lurid colors, ranging from a light purple to a deep blue, so deep it appeared black. Black and blue.

Gently and slowly, I sponged his body with warm water and soap, taking care to dry each part before going on to the next so he wouldn't catch a chill. I talked to him as though we were relaxing at home. "It's Tuesday, Gerry. You're in the hospital because you were in a motorcycle accident Saturday night. If we were home, you'd be taking out the garbage."

I verbally painted a picture of our daily activities, hoping to trigger some response. And it did. After commenting on what our children probably had done that day in school, Gerry voluntarily turned his head towards me, and opened his mouth and in a sing song voice said, "Ah, Ah, Ah, Ah." He didn't open his eyes, but his eyebrows moved up and down to emphasize what he was telling me. It made me cry. Kissing his forehead, I said: "I know dear. I know." I felt quite confident in his progress when I left that night. He looked and sounded so much better.

My confidence was dashed the next morning. The nurse greeted me at the door to say Gerry had developed a severe case of pneumonia. They had him propped up to ease his breathing. I was angry nobody had called me. The staff had promised to call if there was any significant change. This was significant! However, this nurse was not the one working the night before and nothing had been marked on his chart to contact me. She reacted as though I was overreacting.

"This is to be expected," she said. "After all, he aspirated blood and vomit into his lungs."

"That may be, but I wasn't prepared for this." If it was to be expected, then why hadn't someone warned me? I'd certainly asked enough questions to indicate I wanted all the information I could get. The tone was set for the day, making it feel longer than usual. Gerry's responses were less than the day before, but he did push the airway out of his mouth and refused to allow the nurse to put it back in. The oxygen eased his breathing so the staff saw no point in forcing him to have the airway replaced. This reversal from the night before angered me. I was angry with God, angry at life, and angry with Gerry for wanting to be a motorcycle officer in the first place.

Dr. Huang arrived at 4:00 p.m. to assess Gerry. I was on pins and needles watching the nurse review the chart with him. Their expressions were very serious. I wondered if the concern was about the depth of his coma as Dr. Huang placed the chart on his bed.

"Gerry, open your eyes. Gerry, you are in the hospital. Open your eyes. Your wife is here to see you. She sure would like to see those blue eyes."

With each sentence, Dr. Huang raised his voice as if the louder he got, the more likely it would waken him. I was frozen as I watched for even the tiniest reaction. Dr. Huang rocked Gerry vigorously back and forth in the bed. Still no response. The doctor looked worried. He and the nurse administered pain stimuli tests and made notes on the chart. I remembered watching those same tests performed on my brother Brian the year before. Gerry's lack of response frightened me.

Dr. Huang and the nurse turned away whispering. I kept my eyes on Gerry hoping the doctor could give me some indication of his concern. They didn't see Gerry move. My eyes widened with excitement! Gerry began to stir. I was so spellbound, I couldn't speak to get their attention. Instead I slapped my hand on the railing and shrieked. It startled them. I pointed at Gerry. He was yawning and yawning, rubbing his stomach just the way he did at home when he had been napping on the sofa. There was no doubt in my mind that he was waking up. Dr. Huang didn't agree, considering the results of their assessments minutes earlier.

"No, please don't leave. He's waking up. I'm sure of it," I pleaded, excitement bubbling inside.

Gerry kept yawning and rubbing his stomach. Then he stretched his mouth wide and let out a loud noise, patting his tummy as if he had just eaten a turkey dinner. I moved closer to the head of the bed, watching him try to open his eyes. The swelling allowed the eyelids to separate only slightly. Nonetheless, they were open.

"See, Dr. Huang! He's waking up. He pats his tummy just like this when he's waking from a nap on the couch." I was so excited! Dr. Huang laughed.

Gerry looked at me. He looked confused. I thought momentarily it was because he had no idea where he was. Then I realized there was more to it. I was confident he could see me, even with his eyes just tiny slits. To be sure, I slowly walked around the bed so his eyes could follow. He didn't take his eyes off me as I circled the bottom of the bed, walking up the other side. At the top, I leaned closer and looked into his eyes.

"Gerry, I can see you and I know you're looking at me. Really, after all this time, the least you could do is say, hi!"

He paused briefly and then bellowed a gruff, "HI!" It was loud enough to attract the attention of visitors and staff. We laughed out loud. He sounded so funny, so emphatic. His voice was deep and scratchy. Nevertheless, the sound lifted my heart. I couldn't stop looking at him.

Gerry began to fall asleep. Dr. Huang explained he'd drift in and out of a coma for the next few days. However, I could be comforted that the danger had passed. Feeling like a teenager in love, I couldn't wait to be alone with my husband. After the doctor and nurse left, Gerry opened his eyes again.

"Hi, Honey," I said, smiling. "I love you." I wanted to hear him say those words back to me. He didn't. He just stared. Something was wrong! My fingers grazed his cheek and I spoke to him again.

"Hi, Honey. It's me, Janelle, your wife."

I held my breath waiting for a response. There was none. Tears filled my eyes.

"Oh, my God, you don't know who I am."

I Don't Want to
See Daddy

My family is quite close. When one of us has a problem, we like to be there to help. Unfortunately, not all my immediate family lived nearby. My eldest sister, Debbie, lived a six-hour drive south, and the next youngest sister, Rachel, was eight hours north in Williams Lake. They were unable to come at the time. The youngest, Natalie, who lives in northern Alberta was the only one from out of town who could get away to be with us. Her flight arrived late on the evening Gerry came out of the coma, so I decided we should go to straight to the motel after picking her up.

In the morning we enjoyed a leisurely breakfast before going to the hospital. That was the first time in five days that I indulged in a decent meal. It wasn't that I didn't feel hungry, it was more that I couldn't stop thinking about Gerry when I wasn't sitting at his bedside. Not even to eat.

As I maneuvered my car down the street in search of an open restaurant, the sun filtered through the windshield and a gentle breeze slipped through the open window. It had been raining for days. The change in weather brought about a much needed change in attitude for me. I couldn't help feeling energetic and full of enthusiasm. Even my fears from the night before, when I lay in bed worrying whether Gerry would know me, didn't seem so frightening. Somehow, he would come around and, when he did, everything would be okay. Or so I hoped!

I was surprised when we entered the hospital and made our way into ICU to see Gerry sitting in a large recliner near the nurses' desk. Slightly slumped forward, he was sound asleep. The nurse caught me glancing at the restraints around his chest and waist and explained it was necessary to tie him into the chair because he was simply too weak to hold himself up. Nor did he realize he was unable to maintain his balance and, should he attempt to stand, he would invariably injure himself.

There was a stool right beside him for me to sit on. Gently I called his name. There was no response. For that, I have to admit I was almost grateful. I was really afraid to face the possibility that he still might not know me. How would I tell him? Would it still matter?

It wasn't long before he lifted his head, resting it against the chair. Then his eyes opened. He looked at me, wordless, silent. He just stared. The swelling in his face and gums still gave him a toothless appearance. The striking red in his bloodshot eyes was a sharp contrast against the white plaster cast on his nose and cheeks.

The flatness in his eyes was haunting. It was almost a hateful look. Was that what he was feeling toward me – hate? Maybe he was angry with me, thinking I was responsible for putting him in the hospital? Whatever it was, it frightened me. My own husband looked like a perfect stranger.

Within minutes he became restless and began to pull at the catheter, then the intravenous line and finally the oxygen mask. As gently as I could, I took his hands away explaining why he shouldn't pull at them. But as soon as I finished talking, he pulled at something else. Finally a nurse came to my rescue as I was trying to divert his attention from the oxygen mask. "He could probably do without that," she said. "He's breathing just fine on his own. All we were doing was trying to keep the bandages moist."

Cautiously she lifted the elastic band that held the mask securely over his head. Gerry glanced upwards ever so slowly as if wondering what she was doing. He didn't resist but instead began tugging at the electrocardiograph patches pasted to his chest. The nurse chuckled.

"Oh, I see. We're playing a little game, are we? Well, you're right. You don't need those on any more either, so I'll take them off too." She pulled up a stool and delicately peeled the white sticky circles away from his skin. Gerry stared at her. Each time a patch pulled the hairs on his skin, he scowled at her. He didn't complain, but she was sympathetic to his reactions.

"Sorry, big guy. I know it pulls. I'll try to be more gentle." Once the final patch was removed, the nurse got up to leave. "There, that should keep you happy for a while."

Wrong! She hadn't left his sight when he yanked with what little

A Change of Mind

strength he had on the intravenous line. Catching his brisk movement in the corner of her eye, the nurse reacted quickly by clamping her hand on top of the tubing so it couldn't move.

"Oh no you don't. Sorry, but this is one you can't win." She called for another nurse to bring an arm restraint. Turning toward me she explained, "I'm going to restrain his right hand, leaving the one with the intravenous free. It may upset you, but trust me it's for his own protection. We don't want him injuring himself further by ripping out something he shouldn't."

"Oh, it's okay," I said. It was the logical thing to do and her instincts were right. But I still didn't like to see it. I felt badly for him, as though he were a helpless child who didn't understand why these things were being done.

As before, he didn't resist. He just stared as one nurse held down his arm and the other loosely tied it to the chair. When they left I sat beside him. He looked around, moving his eyes slowly, as though he didn't know where he was. I spoke softly to him, explaining again that he had been in an accident and was in the hospital. He ignored me, then drifted off to sleep. It was a good opportunity to make some phone calls and grab a cup of coffee.

When we returned Gerry's nurse greeted me with a smile, the kind of smile when someone knows something that you don't.

"What?" I curiously asked.

"Oh, I think you'll notice a big difference in your husband since you left."

"I've only been gone about twenty minutes. What possibly could have happened since then?"

Her laugh echoed through the quiet room. "Take a look for yourself." It was baffling at first to see what she was talking about. There he was. Still sitting in the chair and awake. He looked the same but then it clicked.

"Oh, my goodness! The cast is off his nose. What happened - did it fall off?"

"Not at all," she replied. "He pulled it off."

"Ouch," I gasped.

"After you left, he was resting quite comfortably so I sat down at the desk with my back to him to do some paperwork. A few minutes later, I heard him moan and turned to see what he needed. His eyes were open and the cast was in his left hand. He was holding it up close to his face and turning it from side to side. It was as though he were trying to figure out what the heck it was."

I could just picture him resembling a small child examining a new object.

"The poor guy," I said. "He really doesn't understand what's happened to him."

"Well, there's nothing to worry about as far as the cast goes. It would have fallen off in a few more days anyway, once the swelling went down. His nose is packed quite solid with gauze so he doesn't really need the cast," she explained. Even with the puffiness below his eyes and the rainbow of colors splashed across his cheeks, he looked much better without the cast.

In the early afternoon, the doctor stopped by to see him. Dr. Huang checked Gerry's eyes and reflexes before listening to his chest and asking him questions.

"Hi, Gerry? Do you know where you are?" There was no reply. "Do you remember being in an accident last weekend? This time Gerry shook his head no. The doctor continued. "Do you know who this is?" He pointed to me.

"Ye…a…h," he said in a shallow tone.

"Who? Who is she, Gerry?" He didn't reply.

"Is this your wife?" Gerry nodded his head, yes. I was so relieved. All my fears of him not knowing me were apparently unfounded.

"What's her name? Can you say her name, Gerry?"

Gerry looked at me briefly, then said: "Bar...bar..ra." I was shattered! He didn't know my name. My husband of fourteen years - and now he didn't even know me.

"Barbara. Is her name Barbara?"

"Ye…a…a…h."   The doctor studied Gerry's chart intensely. It documented his family history including my name. "That correct? Is your real name Barbara?"

"No, it's not." I said, shaken.

"Middle name?"

"No, my middle name is Marie."

"Mother's name, then?"

"No, no - there is no Barbara. Not in either family. I don't know any Barbara. To the best of my knowledge, neither does he." I was exasperated. It just didn't make any sense. The doctor didn't comment. Instead he handed Gerry's chart to the nurse and walked away.

A transformation was taking place with Gerry over the course of that day and it left me feeling quite exhausted. I was bouncing between relief, frustration and fear. Each time I made contact with Gerry, either verbally or physically, it was a guessing game how he would react. Sometimes he just looked at me in a state of confusion when I spoke. Other times it was with an expression of disgust.

It was always me who reached for his hand. He never reached for mine. I waited patiently for even the tiniest sensation of a squeeze in acknowledgment of my presence. But he offered nothing. It was so unlike him. Generally he was very sweet and affectionate. Probably the most hurtful thing was that he had no reaction whenever I left. It didn't seem to matter to him when I left or when I came back.

Like wind changing course, so did his mood by nightfall. He was now aggressive and extremely vulgar. All of a sudden he was swearing at the nurses, the visitors walking by, and at me. It was humiliating to witness his poor and inappropriate behavior. There was no other way to describe it. I was embarrassed for me and for my family who were standing by and listening to this. And I was embarrassed for him. In all the years I'd known him, Gerry had been nothing less than a gentleman. Certainly, he enjoyed his fair share of locker room jokes, but he always drew a line in my presence. That was all gone now. I wanted to explain to people around us that he wasn't like this normally. He just wasn't himself.

The evening nurse took control, suggesting very strongly that we go for a leisurely dinner, and then go back to the motel for a good night's rest. It sounded good, but it was difficult to leave. I felt so responsible for him. I tried to convince her that it wasn't necessary for me to go. However, within minutes, Gerry's behavior made my mind up for me.

Natalie and my mother were standing across the bed from me. I went to the foot of the bed and extended my arms on both sides of Gerry's feet and leaned forward. He lay there with a silly grin on his face, the kind of grin when there's an inside joke. I ignored the mischievous look. I explained that the nurse wanted me to leave early and asked how he felt about that. Instead of answering me, as I hoped he would, he lifted a foot and kicked me in the chest. I pretended not to notice and hoped no one else did either. It was silly not to move. I stayed in the same position. Seconds later, he kicked me again. Harder this time. Hard enough to hurt. Hard enough to push me backwards away from the bed.

"What are you doing, Honey? Why'd you kick me?" I asked, almost afraid of the answer.

"I'm playing with those big tits!" he bellowed. Each word echoed loud and clear throughout the crowded unit. How humiliating! My head felt like a sponge. I didn't know what to say, what to do, or even where to look. The expression on my face must have been worth a thousand words, because the nurse was quick to interject.

"This is very a normal thing when people have brain injuries. They display what we call disinhibitions. It means they act out with inappropriate behavior or responses. I know it's hard for families to hear them talk this way, but it is not unusual, really. We are quite accustomed to it."

Wow! For the first time, someone – and someone with training – was offering me information to help me understand where Gerry was coming from. No doubt, it would have been helpful had someone told me about disinhibitions prior to his waking up, so I could have been prepared. Instead, I had been battling embarrassment for his behavior, guilt for my feelings of embarrassment and humiliation. Oddly, I could handle strangers witnessing his bizarre behavior. We'd probably never cross paths again. But my family would always remember.

It was obvious right then and there that it was best I leave early. I knew I needed some time to think things through. I wasn't certain where to begin. But I had to start facing reality, figuring out what I was going to do.

It wasn't easy to figure anything out. My thoughts were consumed with what could happen the next day should his mood remain the same. My sister, Rebecca, and our friend Margaret Ashley were planning to bring our daughters to the hospital. Part of me rationalized that the sooner the girls saw their Dad the better. The other part of me wanted to protect them from being exposed to his crude behavior. Now I had mixed emotions. Would he be any different in the morning? And if he were, would he be worse, instead of better?

Both Myriah and Dale had expressed some fear over the telephone about seeing their Dad. It wasn't easy for me to assuage those fears either. They intuitively knew more than they should. I couldn't tell them what he was like, because that would really frighten them. Then again if I didn't prepare them, it could be equally devastating.

I didn't know for certain what to do, except to be at the hospital early enough the next day so I would be there before they arrived.

The next morning, I went to the Head Nurse for a first hand report hoping to hear anything different about his behavior than I already knew. She said Gerry had had a comfortable sleep with one exception. During the night, the nurse noticed a piece of blood stained gauze sticking out of his mouth. Upon examination, and to her horror, she found it was the surgical packing from inside his nose. Apparently, he had pulled it out, put it in his mouth and then gone back to sleep. It was amazing he hadn't choked on it.

Gerry watched me speaking to the nurse. He didn't call for me nor did he react when he saw me. Natalie, who is a younger, smaller version of me, was with me. We walked to the bed, smiling and saying "Good morning" with hopes of sparking some reaction from him. Natalie knew Gerry had told the doctor my name was Barbara, so she quizzed him.

"Do you know who this is?" she asked, pointing toward me.

"Yeah," he said, keeping his eyes fixed on her.

"Who? Can you tell me her name?" It was nerve wracking waiting for him to answer. I didn't really like her questioning him. It almost felt as if we were both being humiliated. In response, Gerry slowly turned his head, gazing sleepily at me.

"Daishowa."

"Daishowa?" Natalie and I said simultaneously. It was exciting! This information was being pulled from somewhere in his brain because Daishowa is the name of the pulp mill in Peace River, Alberta, where Natalie's husband works. Gerry's subconscious had connected the name to Natalie. Her presence had jogged his memory. There was no point telling him that he had made a mistake, because he couldn't comprehend what he'd said. So I chattily changed the subject.

"Did you remember the girls are coming to see you today, Honey?"

"Girls? What girls?"

"Our girls, Myriah and Dale. Do you remember them? Myriah has long red hair, and Dale has long dark hair."

Gerry stared into space, as though he hadn't heard a word I said. I tried again, but this time with something different.

"Do you know what your name is?" I said, cupping his chin in my hand to turn his head, so he had to look at me. A strange voice came from his mouth. It shocked me.

"Yes, my name is Christopher Lloyd and I live at 457 Hart Street, England," he said in a crisp British accent with each word pronounced clearly and precisely. Natalie and I looked at each other in bewilderment. Where was this coming from? We had never been to England nor did we know anyone by that name. We certainly didn't have any relatives by the name Lloyd. What really amazed me was his crystal clear voice. When I moved my hand away, he closed his eyes and went right to sleep, totally unaware of what he had just said.

We left him to snooze and waited downstairs in the lobby for Margaret, Rebecca, Myriah and Dale. We had just made ourselves comfortable when they arrived. I was so happy to see them. It had been only six days, yet they seemed slightly changed from when I stopped at Bob and Ruth's the night of Gerry's accident to break the news. In all honesty, they were changed by the events over the past few days. There was no doubt I was, too.

We decided to take the girls to lunch and have a visit first, before going to see Gerry. Both were full of chatter, briefing me on their schooling and how the Ogdens were doing.

"Mom, you wouldn't believe what you did!" said Myriah, waving a small hand before me.

"Me? What did I do, Honey?"

She started to laugh. Laughing so hard she was holding her tummy.

"What? What's so funny?" I asked.

" Remember Dale - the clothes?" Myriah waved to her sister to get her attention.

Dale grinned and started giggling too. "Oh yeah, Mom. Our clothes."

"Your clothes? What about your clothes? I dropped them off to you before I left."

Wiping a tear of laughter from the corner of her eye, Myriah leaned forward with her elbows on the restaurant's checkered tablecloth.

" Yeah, and not a thing fit us. Where did you get them - from the basement?"

"What are you girls talking about? I got them from your dresser."

"Mom, everything you packed for us was way too small. Mr. Ogden had to take us to Naramata so we could get stuff for school," Myriah said emphatically.

I was surprised. Surely I must have looked at what I was taking. Then I began to laugh, remembering what I'd done with my own things.

"You know, I guess it's possible because I decided to have a shower after we checked into the motel. Naturally I needed a change of underwear. What a shock when I went into my suitcase! I took everything apart, searched all the compartments, and sure enough I couldn't find any. What I did find though was every slip I owned - black, blue, white, pink. Long slips, short slips, full slips – you name it – I had it all."

Everybody laughed some more until a cheerful and recognizable voice interrupted us.

"Hi there!"

My children, who were sitting across from me, shrieked with excitement. "Wendy!" they cheered.

Pushing back the leather chair I turned to see our friends, Bob and Wendy Monahan from Quesnel. Wendy had called late the night before saying they couldn't stay away and were leaving early the next morning. Our families had met eleven years earlier when Gerry and I moved two doors down from them. They also have two daughters. Tammy, the eldest, was our first babysitter and Leigh Ann took over when Tammy was too old for babysitting. We had merged our families together over the years including our parents, brothers, sisters, even aunts and uncles. There had not been a time when our families did not share in the good and bad. This time was no different.

The waitress came to take meal orders and refill coffee cups.

"Must be a family reunion," she commented.

"Well, not exactly," I said. "But the next best thing."

It was about this time that my ten-year old astounded me with some thoughts she must have been having over the past few days. She sipped at her chocolate milk and wiped her hand across her upper lip before rattling off several questions and statements.

"Mom, who is paying for all these medical bills you're racking up?" she asked. "I sure hope the RCMP are going to help you. After all, if Daddy hadn't been working, then he wouldn't have gotten hurt. They should accept some responsibility, too!"

"Oh, Honey, of course they will. Don't you worry. We have extended medical coverage. Anything Daddy needs that is not covered under the regular insurance will definitely be paid for by the force."

"Good!" she replied, giving her head one sharp nod as if to say, "That's the way it should be."

The waitress arrived, balancing two meals on one arm and a meal in each hand. She placed beef dips, burgers, and salads on the table and then retreated to the kitchen for a second load. We were all starved. Over the past few days we learned to eat when we could. Often it would be too late when we left the hospital to find some place even to get a sandwich.

"Mom, can we stay here with you?" asked Dale.

"Well, I don't know, dear."

"Please, Mom, could we?" added Myriah.

"If you want Janelle, I can come back up to get them tomorrow," offered Margaret. That would solve my problem. I had no idea how much longer I'd be in Kelowna. Keeping them indefinitely out of school wouldn't be wise.

"Well, okay. There's lots of room in the motel unit. You girls can sleep with me. Grandma and Aunty Natalie can have the hide-a-bed."

When we arrived back at the hospital, I went into the unit to see how Gerry was doing and to inform the staff that I'd be bringing our children in one at a time to see their Dad. There was only one nurse at the station who was talking on the telephone. She made notes and casually glanced up at me. It struck me as odd that I had never seen her before. As if to indicate she would be right with me, she held a singular finger in the air. It indeed was only seconds before she hung up the phone.

"You must be Mrs. Breese?"

"Yes, I am. I just wanted …" Before I could finish my sentence the nurse interrupted.

"Just a second, please. I need to discuss something with you." My eyebrows pulled together, as I waited for what I assumed would surely be information on Gerry's condition.

"The hospital switchboard has been flooded with telephone calls regarding your husband."

"Yes, I know. The nurse this …"

"I know the nurse on shift this morning discussed it with you. She noted you'd select a liaison between your family and the police station to relay any updates on his condition. We must insist you follow through with this. We can't possibly keep answering calls about him. We are very busy here."

She handed me a list of names from callers that morning. The hair on the back of my neck stood up. How dare she assume I had not done what I said I would! Furthermore, how was I to stop people from calling!

"Excuse me," I said. "If you'd let me explain. I *have* appointed a liaison for the family and the police. First of all, it's going to take a while before word gets around, and second, from this list I can tell you right now these people don't even live in the Okanagan. All of them are people we've met over the years in various postings. If they don't know about a liaison then, quite frankly, I can't help it."

The nurse ran a hand through her blond hair, nervously tapping her pen on the desk. "Oh … well, I can see your point about people from out of town. Part of the problem is the media. We know your husband has only one living brother. This morning, we received two inquiries from women who claimed to be his mother and sister."

I was totally shocked. Who would do such a thing?

"We believe it was probably the media. They have been hounding us for an update. We told them they would have to obtain the information from a family member."

"I guess it shouldn't surprise me," I said. "Let's face it, a police officer listed in critical condition is considered a newsworthy story. What I can do is have Inspector Thompsett release a statement about Gerry's present condition and that he has been upgraded. I suppose once they find out he isn't going to die they won't be interested anymore."

The nurse raised her eyebrows, obviously somewhat taken back by my statement, "I guess you're right, bad news is the only good news

A Change of Mind

as far as selling papers go."

Changing the subject, I explained to her that our children were waiting outside to see their Dad. I suggested that perhaps a nurse would like to come and speak to them first. She agreed, and followed me out into the waiting area.

Both the girls were huddled together on a leather sofa. Their hands were tucked on their laps, their hair combed in exactly the same style, wearing matching outfits. The nurse assumed they were twins, a mistake often made by strangers. She took the next 20 minutes to explain in detail what the children would see when we took them into the unit. She described the equipment, how many patients were in the same area as their father, how Gerry looked, and even what he might say when he talked to them. In terms understandable to a child, she described how he had a big bruise on his brain and it would take time to heal.

I watched as our daughters sat, not moving a muscle, taking in every word the nurse said. Both girls shook their heads when asked if they had questions letting their silky bangs wisp gently across their foreheads. Myriah's chin lowered and her eyes became misty when I said I would take her in first. When I took her by the hand, she pulled back and began to cry.

"No! I don't want to see Daddy! I'm scared!"

"Please, Myriah," I pleaded. "I'll be right beside you. It's really important for you to see Daddy … he needs you."

"No-o-o," she sobbed.

Now what? I didn't blame her, but I knew deep down after they saw him they would feel better.

"How about you, Dale? Do you want to go in to see Daddy first?"

She began to cry too. The nurse tried again to ease their fears, confirming my thoughts that the quicker the girls saw their father and faced their fears, the better it would be. It took a while but eventually the girls agreed to go in, one at a time. Each time, as I rounded the corner with one of the girls, Gerry spoke to her right away and called her by name. It was shocking to me that he was able to retrieve this accurate information from his brain, when so many things, like my own name, had consistently been incorrect over the past 48 hours. However, it was heartwarming to see some sparkle in his eyes when he recognized his children. His response immediately put the girls at ease.

In a way, I wasn't surprised that the information about his babies surfaced so strongly. He was an excellent father, participating from their births in their day-to-day care and doing his fair share of night feedings and diaper changes. As the girls grew, he remained involved in every aspect of their lives, from Girl Guide Camp to walking the creek beds with them so they'd catch a glimpse of the Kokanee fish going upstream in spawning season. His children meant everything to him, and I knew they'd be his inspiration to fight to regain control of his life.

It was after supper before the girls first saw Gerry's unusual behavior. The three of us had gone into the ICU to say goodnight. I hoped by going in together we would stir some family nostalgia in him. He was once again sitting in the large recliner. His eyes were closed, but he obviously wasn't sleeping too soundly as he opened them when we came closer. Right away he spoke in the same exaggerated British accent as he had earlier that day.

"Hell-lo, hell-lo, hell-lo!!!" Myriah and Dale were surprised and began to giggle.

I didn't want to draw any more attention to this behavior than necessary, so I gave the girls a simple explanation of how he seemed partial to this accent. We should act as though it were normal. I pulled up three chairs for us, forming a semicircle in front of him so he could see us.

"Honey, isn't it nice the girls came from Penticton to see us?" I asked, hoping to start a conversation with him and the kids.

He raised his eyebrows, and lifted one hand while speaking again in a British accent. "Penticton! Well! Snotty! Snotty! Snotty!"

Myriah and Dale covered their mouths and snickered.

"Well, how did you ride?" he continued.

"Margaret Ashley, one of our friends gave them a ride. Do you remember Margaret, Gerry?" I asked, as the girls sat staring at him.

"Oh, Ma-a-ar-ga-ret! Well! I never…!"

The girls suddenly stopped giggling. He was getting louder and louder. The other visitors were beginning to stare. I took a hand from each of the girls, holding them tightly in my lap.

"Yes. I have a pool and a hot tub at the motel so the girls came up to spend the night with me." I smiled at the kids, trying to imply this wasn't so bad.

Gerry's eyes flashed open as wide as the swelling allowed. Anger seethed from them. He tried to grab at me as he yelled.

"A pool! And a hot tub! Fine! Pack your things and get out of my face!" He looked away from us and moved his lips as if he were muttering under his breath. This cut the girls to the bone. Hurt washed over their little faces. This wasn't their Dad! What was happening? Myriah's lower lip quivered as she bit down on it. Dale grabbed my arm, squeezing her cheek against my shoulder. I didn't know what to say. Gerry realized we weren't leaving.

"Go on! Get out! Get out of my FACE!!!!"

Now it was I who fought back the tears. He loves us, I told myself. How can he be reacting this way? Both our daughters got up to leave. I motioned for them to stay, hoping this would pass, that the night wouldn't end for them with this memory.

"No, Mommy! Please, let's go. I'm scared."

I couldn't speak. Tears welled in my eyes. Poor kids. What could I say? Myriah gave my hand a little tug. I stood up and gently patted Gerry's shoulder, afraid to kiss him goodbye for fear of his reaction. The girls walked gingerly past him and suddenly, as if the winter had ended and spring had brought a full bloom of flowers, his mood changed and he called his children.

"Hugs! Hugs! Kiss! Kisses!"

Myriah and Dale hesitated.

"It's okay. Go on. He wants you to … just give him a little kiss."

Softly they kissed his cheek, one at a time, and then hugged him ever so lightly as if they feared hurting him. He waved a hand as we walked through the doors and down the long corridor out of the Intensive Care Unit. I kissed each girl on her forehead, praising them for being so brave.

"Mommy, will Daddy get better?" asked Dale.

"Yes, he'll get better. But there may be some things that are different about him."

"I don't want anything different, I want my old Dad back!" she sobbed.

From One Extreme to the Other

Within 48 hours there was a complete turn of events. Initially, I was told Gerry would be in the Kelowna hospital for several weeks. But now that he was out of a coma, he was considered to be out of danger and the staff felt reasonably secure about moving him. The decision to transfer him back to Penticton actually came as a relief to me. My expenses had exceeded well over four hundred dollars for that week alone. In Penticton, our friends and family would be able to visit him on a regular basis. And instinctively, I hoped the familiar surroundings would help improve his memory. Foremost, it would be far better for our daughters to have us in our own home so they could get back into a routine and feel some sense of security.

Having Gerry in our local hospital was, for me, a signal he was one step closer to coming home. This was both exciting and terrifying. The thought of providing care for him on a long-term basis was overwhelming. For three years, Gerry and I had watched Bob Ogden expend every bit of energy he had to keep his family together as Ruth recovered from her brain injury. The strain on their lives had been phenomenal. There was little doubt in my mind that our family life would be any different.

How would we manage? It meant surrendering our life as we knew it to make room for doctors, physical therapists, and occupational therapists. And of course, there were lawyers for the dreaded court battle.

Nathan and I arrived at Penticton Regional Hospital about one hour after Gerry's arrival by ambulance. He was admitted under the care of our family physician, Dr. Peter Quandt, and the local neurologist, Dr. David Novak - two very fine doctors. We didn't have to look far for either of them. As we entered the hospital, I could see Dr. Quandt talking with a clerk at admissions. The sound of my high heels clicking on the tiles interrupted their conversation.

"Oh, Mrs. Breese. How are you?" he said looking up.

"Mr. Davies," he added nodding his head to my brother who was also a patient of his.

Dr. Quandt directed us to a nearby leather sofa. "Your husband has been admitted and been taken upstairs. I received your message requesting a private room for him. I fully agree with your reasoning on this. However, he's not ready to be on his own unsupervised. As soon as he arrived, he was admitted to a medical floor but he's very hyper and he keeps trying to climb out of bed. I don't feel the nurses can cope with him right now. He really needs one-on-one supervision, so I've moved him to Intensive Care."

Dr. Quandt stood up straight, resting a foot on the edge of the chair and balancing a clipboard on his knee. He hesitated for a moment and gazed out the large plate glass window. "To be perfectly honest, Mrs. Breese, I don't think he should have been transferred back to this hospital yet. He really isn't ready. Did Dr. Huang say why they wanted to transfer him so soon?"

"Actually," I replied, shrugging my shoulders, "I didn't see Dr. Huang. The head nurse told me she was recommending he be transferred back here. She felt he was out of danger and apparently they needed the bed." Suddenly, I now pondered the decision-making of his transfer. Had the neurologist made the decision? Or was it the Head Nurse? And really, who should be making those decisions?

"Well, we will have to make the best of it," said Dr. Quandt, raising his thick eyebrows. "Dr. Novak will be in charge of Mr. Breese's care. But if you have any questions or need me, just call." Dr. Quandt flashed a smile and dropped his foot to the floor and gave me a fatherly tap on the shoulder. "I'll be in to see him on a regular basis too," he added reassuringly.

Nathan and I stood up and each shook Dr. Quandt's hand and thanked him for his time and concern. Then we excused ourselves and headed upstairs to the ICU. Upstairs, I rang the intercom buzzer on the wall just outside the ICU doors and waited for a nurse to answer. Any fear I had of being unwelcome was quickly put to rest. Instead of a voice coming over the intercom, a nurse came out to get us. She greeted us with a smile as if she knew who we were and as if she had been waiting for us to arrive. I was very moved when she told me she had met Gerry several times through work and how sorry she was that our family was going through such a difficult time. Instantly, I felt he was among friends. She walked us inside the unit and pointed to a large corner room with heavy pink curtains drawn across glass doors.

"Your husband is in there, Mrs. Breese. You can go in. Dr. Novak is with him. He has been waiting for you to arrive so he can ask you some questions."

Gingerly I pulled the curtain back. A nurse was checking Gerry's blood pressure. A man whom I assumed to be Dr. Novak observed the procedure as Gerry tried to pull his arm away. The nurse gave us a warm smile when I introduced my brother and me to her and Dr. Novak.

"Hi, Honey," I said, leaning over the bed rail and kissing Gerry's cheek.

He turned his face away and looked out the window. Almost as though he were another person, Gerry began speaking with the fake British accent, "Hell-lo! Hell-lo! Hell-lo!"

Dr. Novak's eyebrows pulled close together. It was obvious to me that this was the first time the doctor had heard Gerry use this voice. I was quick to offer an explanation.

"He's been talking like this off and on since coming out of the coma. Every once in awhile he will say his name is Christopher Lloyd and that he lives at 457 Hart Street in England," I explained.

Dr. Novak looked puzzled. "Is there any connection for him in England, say perhaps relatives?"

"No. I'm completely bewildered by it," I responded.

Dr. Novak picked up Gerry's chart and began writing. Gently he tapped my husband on the shoulder to get his attention. Gradually Gerry turned his head and raised his eyes to look at the doctor.

"Gerry, I'm Dr. Novak. I'm a neurologist. You've been in an accident. Do you know where you are?"

"Yeah, I'm in Edmonton. At the Edmonton Club."

"No, you're not in Edmonton. You're in Penticton. In the hospital."

Silence blanketed the room.

"Where do you work?" asked Dr. Novak.

"I'm unemployed."

"No, you're not unemployed, Gerry. Are you a policeman?"

"No! I'm a mechanic," Gerry sharply replied, glaring at Dr. Novak as if he were highly insulted by the suggestion of being a police officer.

"Do you know who this is?" he asked, pointing at me.

"Yeah." Gerry glanced toward me and then lifted the bedsheet to cover his face. The message was he had had enough of the doctor's questions. I folded back the sheet and smiled at him. He stared at me with a vacant look.

"Is this your wife, Janelle?" continued Dr. Novak.

"Yeah, my wife Lanelle," he answered, seemingly unaware of mispronouncing my name.

Dr. Novak asked Gerry his age, my age and the ages of our children. He replied that I was 14 and he was 12, and our children were 16 and 18.

Like a small boy on a visit to the doctor's office, he reached for the stethoscope wrapped around the doctor's neck. Dr. Novak handed it to him. Gerry curiously examined the metal instrument. When Gerry plugged the stethoscope into his ears, Dr. Novak turned his attention to me. He needed to know if I had noticed a decrease in Gerry's thirst or appetite. He didn't eat very much and he would drink if I gave him something, but I honestly didn't recall him asking for anything over the past few days. Dr. Novak explained that the appetite center of Gerry's brain might have been affected. This center was responsible for all desires within oneself. When working properly, it sent messages of thirst or hunger. It also, he warned, controlled Gerry's desire for sex. Without it working, Gerry might lack in all these areas. Once again, only time would tell.

It bothered me when conversations danced around Gerry. I wanted him to be included so I removed the earplugs of the stethoscope and asked him a question that I quickly came to regret.

"Gerry, are you hungry?" He didn't respond. "Honey, Dr. Novak wants to know if you would like something to eat?" I added.

"Eat? What would I like to eat?" His blue eyes stared straight ahead. He gently patted his tummy before flashing a huge smile at Dr. Novak. "How about some dark pussy! Yeah! Yeah!" he whooped.

There is no way to describe the embarrassment I felt. My immediate reaction was to apologize, but somehow I couldn't. My eyes fell to the floor. Why was this happening? When would it stop? When I looked up, Gerry was staring coldly into space. His hand stretched out in the air to close his fingers around the dust particles floating in a ray of sunshine hovering above the bed. Only seconds had passed, yet he was completely unaware of what he had just said. I turned to Nathan who was facing the window. His hand was clamped over his mouth. His hear no evil, see no evil routine confirmed that I had indeed heard what I thought I'd heard.

"What did he say?" asked Dr. Novak in disbelief.

"I can't repeat it. Trust me, he said what you thought he said." I patted my cheek to cool the fire burning beneath the surface.

Dr. Novak rebounded quickly, beginning to explain Gerry's injury which he said consisted mainly of a contusion or a "big bruise" on the frontal lobes of his brain. This would affect his personality and emotions. Hopefully, his current behavior would be temporary. Dr. Novak confirmed what the nurse had explained earlier about disinhibitions. Gerry had no control over his vulgarity and aggressive behavior. There was hope that in time it would correct itself. Dr. Novak assured me, as did the nurse, that this behavior was very common with brain injuries and often could be worse. Finally, he said Gerry had sustained some permanent brain damage but it was impossible to say just how much.

"How long do you think he will be in hospital?" "Well, Mrs. Breese, we really have to wait and see how he progresses. But, four to six weeks would be a reasonable goal."

"What about his job?" I asked. "Will he be able to go back to work?"

"Oh, yes. I'd say that in about six months he should be capable of returning to work. This will allow plenty of time for the swelling in his brain to reduce."

I was surprised and confused. Was he saying Gerry could return to work as a police officer? Ruth Ogden had been unable to return to any type of work following her accident, a result of her inability to deal with stress. A police officer's job is extremely stressful and I couldn't foresee that Gerry, given his present condition, would be able to cope as he had before. I expressed my concern to Dr. Novak.

"Well, I didn't say he could return to work as a police officer," he clarified. "I do anticipate him being able to return to some type of employment. Now whether that's on the street as an officer, or inside the office at a desk job, is something we will have to determine at a much later date."

I started to ask, "How much later?" Dr. Novak quickly raised a hand to caution me about being premature. I knew he was right. Besides, it certainly didn't appear to be an immediate concern for Gerry. He couldn't even comprehend that he was a police officer. It would do little good for me to complicate matters. I had to trust that as Gerry's abilities returned, Dr. Novak would give serious consideration to him returning to work.

Before leaving, Dr. Novak said he would be ordering tests to determine the amount of swelling in Gerry's brain. A contusion needs to be assessed regularly. Sometimes a shunt is put into the patient's brain to help ease the swelling and pressure. In Gerry's case, the doctors were confident the swelling would reduce naturally and this extreme measure wouldn't need to be taken.

I casually walked Dr. Novak out into the hallway. As soon as he was gone, I realized how incredibly tired I felt. My legs didn't want to move. My arms felt like rubber. There was a chair in front of the curtained window outside Gerry's room so I sat down, resting my head against the glass. My eyes closed as I listened to the sounds around me. There were call bells buzzing, telephones ringing, and cushioned

A Change of Mind

footwear scooting about the floor. I opened my eyes to see two nurses in pastel uniforms pushing a bed with an elderly woman in it. One guided the bed, while the other directed an intravenous pole. The woman was very still, making no sound. The two nurses chatted.

Suddenly, Gerry's voice sent a string of profanity echoing through the ICU. An older gentleman came out from a patient's cubicle just as Gerry yelled that he was going to piss all over the nurses because they didn't stop to talk to him. The man looked shocked and annoyed, as if to say who could be so rude and why would the staff allow such ill mannered behavior from a patient? I was embarrassed. Again, I wished I could explain. Instead, I decided to play the ostrich. I leaned back, closed my eyes and pretended I hadn't heard a thing.

Over the next two weeks, Gerry's emotions went from extreme highs to extreme lows. It wasn't the mood changes that frightened me; it was the deep seething anger towards me that was so unsettling. I couldn't understand why he behaved so abusively towards me. The more coherent he became about his surroundings, the angrier he got. He left me feeling like he thought I was responsible for him being in the hospital, although it wasn't clear to me that he really knew where he was. He just didn't seem to like it.

Looking back, it seems so odd that I stayed at the hospital from 8:30 in the morning until at least 9:00 each evening and, that in all that time, I had very little interaction with the medical staff. While the nursing staff came in and out regularly to take his vital signs, they did little to enter into a conversation with me. No one mentioned his often shocking behavior and profanity. Surely they could hear him yelling "F-this… F-that!" The ward wasn't large and his door was never closed.

I listened to his offensiveness and watched him slobber and hallucinate. I was at a loss to understand how the staff could make an in-depth assessment if they didn't actually spend any length of time with him - or that matter, if they didn't even at least ask me any questions. The only conversation that sticks out in my mind throughout his first two weeks at the Penticton hospital was a confrontation I had with the Head Nurse of the ICU. Believe me, this altercation did not work to increase my confidence in their assessments of his condition.

It happened shortly after lunch one day. She suddenly appeared in the doorway and called me aside. We stepped outside Gerry's room. "Mrs. Breese, I noticed you were spoon feeding your husband his soup," she began with a very principal-like tone. "We understand families need to mother the patients, but we must insist you let your husband feed himself." Her condescension grated like fingernails on a blackboard. How dare she treat me like a child!

"Yes. You're right! I was feeding him," I responded, curtly. My voice escalated to a level of sharpness which surprised even me. "What do you expect? He's served soup in a bowl which must be eaten with a spoon." I paused momentarily. "Take a look at him. His left hand is immobilized with the intravenous and his right hand, which I might add is the hand he normally uses to feed himself, has a cast on it because his thumb is shattered." I leaned forward and actually bellowed, "HE CAN'T HOLD A SPOON TO EAT!" The rage in my voice halted the activity in the hallway.

Tears of humiliation welled in my eyes. I hated this place! I hated what was happening to us! If she thought I was doing it wrong, why didn't the staff take the time to look after him? God forbid, I thought, if I had not been with him when his food arrived no one would have bothered to feed him. The kitchen staff would just take his tray away at the end of the lunch hour, no one bothering to even notice that he had been unable to fend for himself. My eyes locked onto the nurse's. The red hue of her cheeks clearly indicated her embarrassment.

"Oh! You have a point. I guess I didn't give much thought to it before speaking." She gazed at Gerry and then added, "Perhaps we can have someone from rehabilitation modify his cast so he can use his utensils."

All indications were that I should expect someone from rehab that day. However, the day went by, as did the next and the next. No one came from rehab. It didn't occur to me that I should, or could, call them myself. It was a difficult position to be in. I wanted to be Gerry's voice, yet I feared overstepping my bounds. I clearly lacked confidence in my right to be his advocate. Instead, from then on, I ordered foods for him that could be eaten with his fingers. If there wasn't a meal on the menu suitable to be eaten that way, I just fed him myself. Ironically, no one mentioned the situation again.

It was a relief when Dr. Novak announced Gerry was coherent enough to be transferred downstairs to a private room. The idea of having some privacy was wonderful. And I was certain the activity level on a regular ward would be less and thus, more relaxing. What a joke!

From the moment Gerry arrived on SP3, total chaos took over. The staff was almost beside themselves trying to deal with him. He was hyper and uncooperative. The most difficult part was he had no concept of where he was, what he should be doing, and what might happen when he did something. Gerry needed constant supervision and the staff was completely unable to provide it - not for lack of skills, but for lack of manpower.

That's when I really had to call upon my family for help. About a week after Gerry was placed on the ward, his sleep patterns became more and more disturbed. His day usually began before dawn, about four o'clock in the morning. The nursing staff requested that I, or someone from my family, come to the hospital by that time to help with him so they could get their work completed before shift change. It was glaringly obvious to me that in cases where there is no family to help out, survivors of a brain injury may not have adequate supervision. There is no volunteer system in place to help out. Caregivers may be funded through insurance or compensation; however, this takes time to put in place and is often months down the road.

My mother graciously took on the job for me. It meant, however, that I had to send a taxi to pick her up by 4:30 a.m. and provide her with the money to pay for it. This cost nearly ten dollars a day because she had to take a taxi home too. I would take the kids to school at eight o'clock and then head straight to the hospital to relieve Mom. I made arrangements for our girls to take the school bus into town after school and I slipped out from the hospital to pick them up. I'd get something for them to eat for dinner at the hospital. We stayed there until after I bathed Gerry and put him to bed usually around 9:00 p.m.

Gerry's memory showed signs of improvement daily. But it wasn't always positive, such as when he remembered he smoked. Having been without a cigarette for two weeks, I was certain he would find quitting easy. But when he recalled that he was a smoker, it was as if he had not been a day without one. He asked everyone for a cigarette - the nurses, the orderlies, even perfect strangers who were walking down the hallway. Because I was with him so much, I had to keep telling him that he couldn't smoke in the hospital. As far as Gerry was concerned, I was the one who was stopping him from smoking. He didn't believe for one second that it was a hospital rule. Maybe it would have helped if he had been given nicotine gum or patches to wear to help with the cravings. Not being a smoker myself, it never occurred to me to ask the doctor about this.

On top of this, Gerry's moods went from high to low. Constantly. It was like a wild roller coaster ride until I was beginning to feel my reactions were out of place. One day in particular stands out in my mind. It was a hot and sticky afternoon. Gerry had been badgering me for a cigarette all day. My unwillingness to cooperate had deeply angered him. He hadn't spoken a kind word to me since morning. In late afternoon, a group of police officers came to visit. Gerry's face lit up like a child on Christmas Eve. I helped him into the wheelchair. He scooted around the room, shaking hands with each one. Gerry still couldn't recall that he was a police officer, but that didn't diminish his happiness to see them. About twenty minutes passed when another visitor arrived, a surgical nurse at the hospital who was also a personal acquaintance of ours from Naramata.

"Hi, Gerry," her voice bubbled through the air.

"Hey!" he replied, wheeling his chair closer to her. I wasn't certain whether he really recognized her or not.

"Hi, Bobbi," I said, hoping to spark his memory.

"I'm just taking a little break," she explained, looking at Gerry. "So I thought I'd come down to see how you're making out."

A sheepish grin flashed across his face. The term "making out" had obviously triggered some memories for him.

"Making out? Come here. I'll show you how to make out," he bellowed. He grasped the hem of Bobbi's uniform and lifted her skirt.

Bobbi reacted quickly by pushing his hand away. My mouth gaped. The officers laughed. No doubt, their laughter was from sheer nervousness and embarrassment but at the time I didn't see that. All I heard was this locker room tittering. What I saw was Gerry reacting as though he were a ten-year old boy with a captive audience.

No sooner had Bobbi removed Gerry's hand than he grabbed the other side of her skirt and tried lifting it up. This time she stopped him before he could make any progress by firmly gripping his wrist. But once again, the room filled with laughter.

I struggled to hide my feelings of anger and hurt. "Why didn't they stop him? Did this seem natural to them?" I asked myself. All I knew was something had to be done to stop this madness. But what should, or could, be done? Of course, I didn't want anyone to think I was overreacting and letting petty jealousy take hold.

Once everyone left, I put Gerry into bed and encouraged him to rest before Judie Johnson arrived with Myriah and Dale. Not for a minute did he close his eyes. Instead he called me names and spit at me. Everything was wrong and my fault. He lashed out at me for not giving him a cigarette, for keeping him in the hospital. I sat in the corner of the room fruitlessly trying to tune out the hurtful words.

The lighthearted sound of our children's voices coming down the hallway was like a breath of fresh air. Gerry's mood always softened and he seemed to perk up whenever the girls came to visit. Today I depended on it. Both girls, clad in sneakers, with backpacks over their shoulders, raced through the doorway and headed straight to their Dad for a kiss. He smiled and patted their backs. The harshness in his face dissipated. He nonchalantly picked up the end of Myriah's waist-length coppery braid and twirled it about. Dale's fingers tapped away on her dad's leg as she tipped a pop can to her lips. Following closely behind them was Judie, her son Steven and my Mom. Gerry glanced at them when they entered the room, but ignored their hellos.

I was sitting on the foot of his bed with my hand resting on the crisp bed coverings that were draped over his feet. Judie leaned against the wall while Mom made herself comfortable in the chair next to her. Myriah, Dale, and Steven plunked themselves down on the tile floor, each opening a bag of potato chips and munching away happily. Mom, Judie and I chatted with the kids about their day in school and plans for the summer holidays. Gerry lay quietly in bed. There was a break in the conversation and a comfortable silence hovered in the room. I watched the children in amazement at the ability they had to adjust to circumstances.

Suddenly, like an exploding bomb, Gerry lifted a leg and kicked me as hard as he could. My hands pushed out to break my fall, but little could stop the force as I landed with a thud on the floor.

"Get out of here! Go on!" Gerry screamed at me, pointing towards Judie. "I don't want you anymore. I want her!"

I didn't want to make a scene, so I got up off the floor and sat on the bed again hoping his mood would shift.

"Honey, it's okay, it's me. Your wife," I soothingly said.

The rage in his eyes was crystal clear. He lifted a foot and kicked me again. This time he kicked me even harder. The kids shrieked when I fell to the floor.

"Go on whore! Get out of here. I don't want you anymore! I want her!" His finger shook in Judie's direction.

I didn't know what to say or where to look. The children's eyes were filled with fear. It was a struggle to get up without bursting into tears. My mind raced with thoughts of the kids having nightmares. While I dusted off my pants, I nodded to the kids.

"Why don't you guys go down to the TV room for a few minutes?" There wasn't an argument from any of them. All three scrambled to their feet and took off. The rest of us stood dumbfounded. By now, I was afraid to get too close to him. We were all thinking if we remained quiet, his mind would go on to something else. Not so!

"You! Get in here!" he hollered to Judie. She shifted from one foot to the other as color painted her cheeks. She nervously tried to divert his attention with small talk.

"Gerry, you know me. Judie. Lloyd's wife. Remember?"

"I don't care. I don't want her anymore." He stared at me coldly.

Judie came over and took my trembling hand. "Look, why don't I take your Mom and the kids out for something to eat? They don't need to see all this."

I nodded my head, knowing that if I spoke the tears would flood forth. I bit down hard on my lip and patted Judie's arm. Mom stopped to hug me. "Maybe you should come too. You need a break, dear," she said.

"No, I have to stay," I whispered.

"Okay, Janelle. But Lloyd's coming here right after work. Promise me that you will go have a cup of coffee while he's here. Let him stay with Gerry," said Judie, with deep concern.

I lowered myself into the chair, nodding in agreement. Seconds later, Gerry and I were in the room alone. Neither of us spoke. I was walking on eggshells with him. Everything seemed to set him off. Half an hour went by before I heard Lloyd's heavy footsteps, echoing down the corridor.

Gerry recognized Lloyd immediately. As his six-foot four-inch, 300-pound frame passed through the doorway, Gerry greeted him by his nickname. "Hey, Tons! Gimme a smoke!"

"Hey, little buddy!" replied Lloyd. "What do ya want to smoke for? Besides, I quit."

"No, you didn't. That box in your shirt sleeve – that's cigarettes." Gerry leaned forward to grab Lloyd's sleeve, nearly falling out of bed.

Skillfully, Lloyd leaned Gerry back into the bed. As he did, the staff brought in a dinner tray. I took the tray and placed it on Gerry's table, rolling it beside his bed and over his lap.

"Here you go, Hon. Hot food!" I said, lifting the steamy metal cover.

"Fuck you!" he shouted giving me a shove.

That was the last straw. I couldn't bear to hear another word. My lip quivered. The metal cover dropped onto the plate.

"Lloyd … Lloyd, can you help him with his dinner? I just have to get some air."

I spun around on my heels and headed for the doorway, not waiting for Lloyd's answer. The tears were pouring by the time I made it to the hallway. The deep sound of my sobs echoed. It wasn't long before someone heard me crying.

"Mrs. Breese, are you okay?" asked the nurse, wrapping her arm around my shoulders. "Do you want to talk?"

"I can't take this anymore. He's so mean to me. It's as though he thinks I'm responsible for all of this."

The nurse smiled sympathetically. "We don't know why this happens. But it seems that survivors of brain injuries lash out as the ones closest to them. You've been here night and day, always keeping a stiff upper lip. It was bound to catch up to you, sooner or later. Let's go into the lounge and have a chat. He'll be okay for a few minutes."

Fortunately the lounge was empty. The nurse sat patiently while I cried, offering words of encouragement. I was emotionally exhausted and remember very little of what she said except that it wasn't my fault and that his reaction to me was not intentional. It was all so hard to understand. He had gone from one extreme to the other in a matter of days. It terrified me to think this may not get any better. Then what?

That night I hardly slept. Flashbacks exploded in my head. It was time to do something I told myself. For if we didn't get some help, there was little chance we'd survive as a family.

A Change of Mind

Homeward Bound

The next morning I was awake by 5:00. As I paced the kitchen floor, I made up my mind that someone was going to have to listen to me today. Every nerve in my body seemed to tremble as I prepared my speech. We needed help.

The hospital hallways were still quiet as I approached Gerry's room nearly two hours later. The girls had stayed with Judie and Lloyd the night before so I decided to take the early shift. A nurse was combing his hair when I arrived.

"Wow, looks like you just got out of the tub," I said pecking him on the cheek. Gerry didn't respond.

"He sure did. Didn't ya big guy?" responded the nurse. There was still no reaction from him.

Uncertain of how to start my speech, I sat down in the chair next to the bed. The nurse made small talk. Very little of what she said sunk in. My mind was wandering, searching for an opportune time to change the subject. "Can I talk to you about something?" I finally asked.

"Sure," she replied.

"Well, first of all, I want to assure you I'm not blaming anyone. Nor am I being jealous. Most of all, Gerry doesn't behave like this usually and I don't want you to think poorly of him." Our eyes met and she smiled. I felt uncomfortable talking about him like this. She sensed my hesitation and encouraged me to go on as if I was a child discovering a new challenge.

"It's okay. Go ahead," she encouraged.

Slowly I went over the events of the previous day. I spared no details, repeating his words and describing his physical abusiveness and how humiliated I felt in front of everyone, especially the guys he worked with.

"You mean to say not one of those guys came to your defense?" she asked, referring to the incident with Gerry lifting the nurse's skirt.

"No, and I really don't blame them. I really don't. I'm sure they were just as embarrassed as I was."

"Well I think it's time you and I have a little chat. Let's go have a cup of coffee. Your husband will be fine for a few minutes. Come on. We'll just be in the lounge."

This was what I wanted – someone who was in charge medically to talk to me about Gerry's behavior. I desperately wanted someone to tell me what to do and how to handle the situation. I wasn't disappointed. Apparently the night shift nurses had had a meeting with the day shift nurses that morning to discuss Gerry's inappropriate behavior towards women. They unanimously believed it was time to take some steps to correct him.

"We were going to explain to you this morning that now was the time to start correcting his behavior," she said.

"But how?" I asked, hoping she'd have some answers.

"Let me explain," she began. "Your husband has lost all his inhibitions. Along with that, he lost his sense of relationships. He doesn't remember, or even understand, what appropriate behavior is. For example, he tried to pull me into the tub with him this morning when I bathed him. While I was drying him, he tried pulling at my uniform. As a team, the night and day nurses have discussed his behavior and decided it was time to talk with you. We want you to understand that it's time we start correcting this behavior."

"I agree. But you do understand he's not usually like this, don't you?" It was difficult not to feel defensive. Gerry was a great guy, they didn't know him like I did.

"Oh, of course we do, Mrs. Breese. Believe me, it would be a lot worse if he were 18 years old. Now all we want to do is gently, but firmly, remind him what is appropriate behavior with women and, naturally, with yourself. One of two things will happen. Either he can learn how to relate to women all over again, or it could take a long time for him to show some changes. Hopefully, after a couple of reminders, something will click in his memory and those boundaries will be reestablished. But of course, we need your cooperation. I assure you, we are not going to be nasty with him. But we do have to be firm."

A Change of Mind

For the first time in days I had something concrete to hold on to. My entire outlook shifted. Somebody was listening. She seemed to understand and I felt we were all working together, working toward the same goal which was ultimately to return Gerry to his previous life.

I discovered, through my conversation with her, that this nurse had sustained a brain injury fifteen years earlier. The fact she had recovered enough to return to her regular position as a hospital nurse gave me tremendous inspiration. Later in the morning, we met again to discuss setting up a support system with family and friends. It was imperative that they too not allow Gerry's behavior to go unchecked.

My first step was to talk with Hughie Winters, my liaison with the RCMP. Both he and Nathan assured me they'd pass the word around to visitors from the office that they shouldn't encourage Gerry's behavior if and when he was inappropriate – especially with laughter.

Later that afternoon another situation occurred when I took him for a jaunt up and down the hallways in the wheelchair. Whenever I did this, he repeatedly tried to get out of the chair and walk. However, his gait was impaired because of the disruption to his equilibrium so he could stand for only seconds before becoming dizzy. As we turned the corner of the nurses' station, an attractive young blonde nurse caught his attention. She was helping an elderly man walk and didn't seem to notice us. It never occurred to me that Gerry had anything in particular on his mind. But he did. I guided the wheelchair alongside the nurse and the man so that we could pass them. As soon as we were within reach, Gerry reached out and slipped his hand underneath the nurse's uniform.

She gasped, as did I. The elderly man didn't notice a thing.

"Excuse, me!" she bellowed, her eyes darting from Gerry to me.

"I'm terribly sorry," I said, blushing. With a deep chuckle, Gerry reached for her again. This time she was prepared.

"Hey, I've heard about you. That's not appropriate. I'm not your wife. You don't even know me," she said, firmly holding Gerry's wrist. "You can't do that to people."

Gerry just looked at her without speaking. Her eyes connected with mine as she released his hand. The sympathy and understanding she seemed to silently convey did little to soothe my feeling of embarrassment. I just wanted all this to stop. I wanted Gerry to be the way he was before the accident. He respected me and he would have never made such advances towards another woman.

It took quite a bit of effort for the nurses to be on top of his actions and for me to gain some backbone and be firm with him. Visiting police officers pitched in and helped too. Whenever Gerry made vulgar comments they reminded him it wasn't appropriate.

Over the next several days Gerry began to show a change in his attitude. The occurrences of him acting inappropriately toward the nurses became less frequent. Then one day he stopped making sexual advances altogether. It was as if something had clicked. This was a good sign.

We were so engrossed with Gerry's emotional status that we were caught off guard when he developed a bladder infection nearly three weeks after the accident. It started with him saying he didn't feel good. He was restless and running a low-grade fever. He complained of having pain when he went to the bathroom, especially around his right testicle. The nurse gave him a hot water bottle and tried to get him to lie on his left side. Gerry found it too painful to put pressure on his left hip which was badly bruised, so he didn't want to lie down or sit for too long. Fortunately, with prescribed antibiotics the infection subsided within a few days.

It was well into early summer and the days were getting hotter and hotter. The hospital air was stale and dry. It seemed natural to start taking him outside for short periods of time. I felt like a caged animal walking the hallways every day, so I could only imagine how he felt.

Finally, I asked Dr. Novak for permission for a day pass so I could take him out of the hospital for lunch or supper. He agreed. We didn't venture too far away. Often our reprieve was nothing more than going outside on the hospital grounds for a soft drink, sandwich and some fresh air. Regardless, each time the doors opened, I breathed deeply filling my lungs with the warm air. It felt like freedom.

However, no matter what the excursion or its length, it was exhausting for Gerry. One night I took him to my mother's for dinner.

This required him to endure a five minute car ride from the hospital to her house. As soon as we arrived, he had to lie down for a rest. A full hour and a half went by before he awoke. When he did, he wanted to leave – immediately.

His wanting to leave abruptly happened frequently. It did not matter if we were only on the hospital grounds or at a restaurant for lunch. Within a minute or two of arriving, he wanted to go back to his hospital room. And if I didn't move fast enough, he got quite vocal about it. It became quite frustrating and costly. I paid for several meals which were left virtually untouched.

Yet overall, his condition – especially his memory — improved steadily. By June 9th, he could recall specific details about articles, events or persons. However, he did not remember getting married, the house we lived in or when our children were born. When I spoke with Dr. Novak about this, he explained Gerry had retrograde amnesia. He could not remember events or people from before his brain injury. He had to visually see something or someone to remember any distinct details like names or events.

After giving some thought to my conversation with Dr. Novak, I decided to be creative. So I brought all our photo albums, including our wedding and the girls' baby books into the hospital. As Gerry flipped through the pages, his face lit up. The names of people and places began to flow from his tongue. The only exception was our house.

He had to see where we lived to remember it. Dr. Novak gave me a pass for an afternoon so I could take Gerry to Naramata. As I stopped the car in our gravel driveway, Gerry's eyes scanned the yard and neighborhood. He couldn't wait to get out of the car. Gerry still had to use a walker or wheelchair, but he wasn't prepared to wait for either this time.

The sun was shining, the flowers were in bloom, and the sound of chirping birds filled the air. I helped him get from the car into the house. It was like Christmas. He wanted to see everything, touch everything. I had to physically help him from room to room as our house was older and not set up for wheelchair access.

"I don't want to go back to that place," he said.

"Where? The hospital?"

"Yeah, I'm staying here."

"Oh, Honey. I know you want to come home, but you have to stay there just a little while longer. Dr. Novak said he wants to wait until your balance is a little better."

The sad look in his eyes tugged at my heart. He wanted to come home. I wanted him home, but looking after him on my own would be overwhelming. However, only three days later I was talking to Dr. Novak about just that. It seemed the logical thing to do even though I had told Gerry otherwise. The girls and I were always at the hospital. When we were there, the nurses left us in charge of his care. I really couldn't see any point in keeping him there. His medication could be administered at home and his need for constant supervision could be handled.

Dr. Novak wasn't that convinced. "I'm not certain you could cope with him at home," he explained. "He doesn't sleep very well, and I think, with the constant disruption in your routine, it won't take long before you become exhausted yourself."

"I'm exhausted now, Dr. Novak," my voice quivered. "My mother comes here at 4:30 in the morning and my day starts here by 8:30. I stay with him until he is in bed at night. There isn't anything he gets here that I can't give him at home."

"I understand that, Mrs. Breese. But my concern is for you. This is a tremendous responsibility."

Tears welled up in my eyes. "Please, Dr. Novak. He wants to go home. I need to try and get him, my children and myself into a routine. He may never get any better and I can't commit our lives to being at this hospital. Besides, he'll progress more quickly in his own surroundings."

"You've got a point," said Dr. Novak, placing a hand firmly on my shoulder. "Okay, let's make a deal. I understand the RCMP is willing to pay any expenses you may incur for his care. You go speak to them. If they agree to pay for a home nurse to help you, then I'll agree to let him go home. How's that sound?"

I sighed. It sounded good, but I knew my own habits. "Dr. Novak, I want to take care of him. I want to care for my children. So I don't think having a nurse in our home would work. However, I don't have a problem surrendering duties like cooking and cleaning. I'll go along with having a non-medical employee who can take over those household duties for me but who is also suitable as a companion for him. That way I can get out to do errands and he'll have the supervision he requires to keep him safe and out of harm's way. Would that work?"

A warming smile came over the doctor's face. "Yes, that would work. But you must have this in place before I'll discharge him. Agreed?"

My instincts were to hug him. I was thankful for his cooperation. It was exciting to know I'd be taking Gerry home. We were one step closer to getting our lives back to normal.

It took two days to make the necessary arrangements. Hughie Winters worked with Inspector Thomsett who in turn got permission for me to hire help with the guarantee the RCMP would pay the person's wages. The one condition was that I pay the wages first and then submit a bill for reimbursement. This would add strain to our financial situation but it would be worth it.

The woman I hired was a long time friend of ours, Marilyn Paine. We had met her when our children were just babies. She was a very spiritual and family-oriented person. This was important, because I needed to have someone I trusted. I had to be assured Gerry would be treated with patience and kindness in my absence. Her starting date was scheduled for one week after Gerry came home. This was to give Marilyn time to make arrangements and also to give the four of us time to adjust. Typically, I thought it would be easier than it was.

It was a beautiful morning the day Gerry came home. The air was fresh, the trees had new buds, and birds were singing their songs of spring. It was the type of day that makes you thankful to be alive. I was twice as thankful.

Our daughters were so excited about their father coming home. They wouldn't miss the long days at the hospital. They needed to get on with their own lives and start being children again. But it wasn't going to be that easy. Our family structure was still out of sync. Gerry's emotional state was far more childlike than our children's. That made it extremely difficult for the girls to relate to him as their father.

What made it even more difficult was the medical professionals kept telling us that the kids and I should just go on being ourselves: the wife, the mother, the kids, and the daughters. They would take care of Gerry. *What they didn't seem to understand was that we couldn't be who we were, because he was no longer who he had been.*

It was difficult to get them to understand why I kept saying it was impossible for me to just go on being the wife and mother. I explained it like this: Consider the cast of a Broadway play. Typically, the same actors and actresses perform in a Broadway production for years and years. There is a leading man and a leading lady. There are supporting characters and extras, all bringing the production together with their contributions. While I am confident these productions have ongoing rehearsals, the longevity of the production enables the cues, lines, and positioning of the cast to become second nature for actors and actresses. But can you imagine what would happen if after ten, twelve or fourteen years, the leading man shows up for work one night and can't remember his lines anymore? He can't remember where to stand, or what cue to give his leading lady. How could the leading lady play her part? It wouldn't matter how great an actress she is. If everyone is not "playing their part" then not only can she not play her part, but no one else can either. Even if they tried, the production itself would make no sense.

Take it a step further. What if the writers, director and producers (the professionals) told her, "Yeah, we know he's changed and can't play the part anymore, but you just go on being the leading lady – you do your part – we'll take care of him." How much sense would that make? None!

That was the exact predicament of our family. Gerry and I had been working at our production for fourteen years. We could, undoubtedly like other couples, anticipate the reaction of our partner in almost any given situation. There were times that I took the lead and there were times that he took the lead. Regardless, each of us trusted that the other would do his or her part.

Now my leading man had virtually traded places with our daughters. It was Myriah and Dale who became equal partners with me in the running of the household and in caring for their Dad. Gerry was now "an extra". I don't say that in a demeaning or bitter way. It was simply the way it was. He no longer had the capacity to contribute as an equal partner in marriage or an equal partner in parenting.

Our life, as we knew it, was gone. Prior to Gerry's brain injury we did everything together-grocery shopping, decision-making, yard work, housework. Everything. I found myself wanting to step back into that routine. But that meant reacting as I always had, sharing everything with Gerry.

He was unable to cope with making even the simplest decision, right down to what he would like for dinner. It became so difficult that eventually, I'd stop when I found myself going to say something to him. Instead of watching him agonize over the smallest detail, it was easier to handle everything on my own. That was a dangerous course for me to be on, but I couldn't see it at the time.

As a father, Gerry was no longer recognizable to the girls. Prior to being injured, he was a fully participating Dad. He changed diapers and took the late night feedings when the girls were babies. As they grew up, he immersed himself fully into every stage of their lives. He took them fishing, hunting and snowmobiling. He volunteered at Brownies, Girl Guides and at school. He shared in educating and disciplining them. He kissed their scrapes and bruises and he always, always put his love for them first.

Since the accident, the girls didn't get any of the nurturing they had before. Not even from me. Sure – I fed them, clothed them, made sure they had their homework done and got off to school everyday. But it wasn't the same. The motions we were going through each day seemed mechanical. For all intents and purposes, these two little girls no longer had either parent. I had nothing left over in the day to be their Mommy, and the Daddy they knew never came back.

There was nothing familiar about him. He even looked different. The 'little-boy' sparkle in his crystal blue eyes was lost and replaced by a flat lifeless gaze. He didn't laugh. He didn't talk to us or with us. And he didn't seem to realize all these things had changed. I missed the old Gerry. I knew the kids did too.

The first few days after Gerry came home, a continuous stream of family, friends and co-workers stopped by to say hello. He was delighted to see them but couldn't relax. He paced back and forth in the kitchen, sat for a minute, and then resumed pacing almost immediately.

Each time someone came to see him, I'd discover something amiss - little things, but potentially dangerous things if not monitored. Late one afternoon Curtis Horton, the "dogmaster" in the RCMP and Chuck Simonin, a local Naramata resident and fellow volunteer fireman, stopped by for coffee. It seemed like only seconds had passed from my filling the coffee cups to Gerry asking for a refill. It surprised me. I refilled his cup and returned to my seat, keeping a skillful eye on him. He picked up the cup of steaming hot coffee and gulped it down in three swallows.

"Honey, isn't that hot?" I asked, my hand clutching my shirt as I imagined the hot sensation going down his esophagus.

"No, just right," he replied.

"It must be hot, buddy," interjected Chuck. "I'm on my first cup and it's quite warm."

"Would you like some more?" I asked. He nodded. Discreetly, I took his cup to the sink, filled it halfway with hot coffee and topped it with cold water. That too, was gone in three swallows.

"How was that?" I questioned.

"The same," he replied.

Curtis raised his dark eyebrows in surprise. "It can't be, Gerry," he said.

"Yeah, it was." It dawned on me that along with his sense of taste, his sensory perception to differentiate between hot and cold was also damaged. It meant that I had to be certain hot foods and liquids were cooled before giving them to him.

"Why hadn't I put two and two together?" I asked myself. The appetite center had been damaged and all along Gerry had complained that his face, lips, tongue and mouth felt numb. Once I figured it out, it made sense to me that he would not be able to determine the difference between hot or cold. But then again, I wasn't certain he understood what I meant by hot or cold.

The revelation that Gerry had to relearn structure and boundaries within his life was painfully obvious. The problem for me was I didn't know where to begin. There had been no list to follow and check off as we came across various situations. I just had to wait for each to occur and hope I could react quickly enough. Unfortunately, there wasn't any reading material on brain injuries to enlighten me. I learned a little more each day and each time we saw the doctor.

A perfect example came the morning after Gerry's first night home. Charged with excessive energy, Gerry's eyes popped open long before the first stream of light filtered through the windows. It wasn't even 4:30 a.m. Tapping me on the shoulder, as though it was his duty to see I got up, he tried to spring from bed. Balance was a problem for him so it took a few bounces back on the bed before he stood solid.

"Honey, it's so early," I said, sleepily.

"Yeah. Lots to do today," he replied.

"Great!" I muttered. Not to him, not to anyone. It was in acknowledgment of my day beginning, knowing there would be no talking him into going back to sleep.

My feet scuffed across the white carpet in search of my fluffy slippers. I pulled my cotton robe over my shoulders. Gerry's voice boomed through the hallway.

"Myriah! Dale! Come on, girls! It's time to get up!" I scrambled to the door as he continued to bellow. "Come on, girls! It's time for school!"

"No! No! Honey." I whispered resting one finger against my lips. "Remember we always – always – let the kids sleep as long as possible. It's not time for them to get up yet. Let's go downstairs and have coffee. Okay? But you've got to be very quiet."

He followed me down the stairs into the kitchen, softly lit from the light on the range hood. After several cups of coffee, I felt reasonably confident in leaving him alone while I indulged in a hot shower. As I toweled off, the heavy silence from downstairs made me curious. It was almost too quiet. As with toddlers – I knew as all mothers do – silence usually means trouble. Peeking down the stairs, I called softly to avoid waking the children.

"Gerry, are you okay?"

"Yeah, great."

"What are you doing?"

"Oh, nothing. Just going for a little ride."

Oh, my goodness! He's going driving! Pulling my robe closed, I scurried down the stairs. There he was, completely dressed: jeans, cowboy boots, western shirt and baseball cap, keys in hand.

I was shaking. My hand quickly gripped the keys, pulling them from his hand. He was still weak from the accident so there was no resistance.

"Why'd you do that?" he asked.

"Because, you're not quite ready to drive. Besides it's only five o'clock in the morning and nobody's up to see you."

His brows pulled tight together. He turned away muttering, heading for the sofa where he plopped down and reached for a magazine. I heaved a sigh as his dirty boots came to rest on the glass coffee table. He glared at me. His anger toward me felt brutal. It cut like a knife. For some time now, there were times when he was very loving toward me and then suddenly, his mood changed drastically.

There was no point in a confrontation so I retreated upstairs to dry my hair. The hum of the hair dryer mesmerized me and my thoughts soon drifted to our life before the accident. As I bent over to unplug the dryer, the bedroom door flew open, startling me. Gerry barreled through, taking long strides, his boots landing with a thud on the floor. A leather jacket had now been added to his ensemble. Sheer determination was carved on his face.

A Change of Mind

"Just going to take a drive down to my brother's," he said. A hand shot past me grasping the keys to our pickup truck on top of the dresser. My hand swiftly covered his.

"Honey, the truck is not insured. Don't you remember?"

"I want to go have coffee with my brother," he insisted.

"I know," I said, soothingly. "But it's way too early. Perhaps after the girls go to school, I could take you down to see him."

"Fine," he huffed, swinging his large shoulders to turn away. "I'm tired. I think it's bedtime."

I stood and watched in astonishment as Gerry peeled his clothes off, each piece landing in a heap on the floor. Before I could even comprehend what was happening, he stretched his naked body out on the bed and drifted off to sleep.

The clock read 5:45. The girls would be up for school in just over one hour, so there did not seem much sense in my going back to bed. Tiptoeing down the stairs, I went to the front room with a fresh cup of coffee.

The sky was awakening, the black lifting to blue. Birds began to chirp. I looked out into the empty street, visualizing that fateful night only weeks earlier when I'd said goodbye to him in the driveway. Exhaustion sent a shiver through me. I pulled the afghan over my legs, sipping at the coffee. "God, how long can this go on?" I whispered out loud. "I just want my husband back. Is that too much to ask for?"

Gerry slept right through the girls having breakfast. It was nice just to know he was upstairs though. Myriah and Dale chatted to each other, showing no signs of what they'd been through. I knew they were happy to have us all home. It felt like an eternity since we had had a normal morning with some routine.

The house wasn't quiet for very long after the girls left for school. I barely had the dishes loaded into the dishwasher when Gerry came downstairs. This time he was dressed in shorts and a T-shirt. Without saying a word, he went out to the back yard. I sat at the kitchen table and peered out over the patio as he strolled across the yard to the creek.

When we originally purchased the house, a lovely wood bridge spanned the creek from our yard onto a small piece of land that was dense with trees and gave the impression of going on for miles. A couple of years after we bought the house, the creek flooded and washed away the trees, our bridge, and nearly six feet of the bank. Now we could see the neighbors' houses behind us and they could see us. It wasn't nearly as beautiful, but we still enjoyed sitting by the creek. The sound of water trickling over the rocks was so serene it was almost hypnotic.

Apparently, that wasn't all the sound of the water did. My eyes were glued to Gerry's large frame as he came to a stop near the edge of the property. His hands rested on his hips as he stared down into the creek. He began to shuffle from one foot to the other, then his hands moved from his hips to the front of his shorts. I gulped as he began to fidget.

"Oh, God. He can't possibly be doing what I think he's doing!" I blurted out to the empty room. I rose from the table, rushing to the patio doors, calling his name. The woman across the creek stood up from her gardening. Her eyes fixed on Gerry as he casually relieved himself into the creek.

Naturally, I overreacted. He had no idea why his actions weren't appropriate. It didn't matter how many times I explained it, he peed in the water every time he went out to the creek that week. Finally, I figured out that the sound of the rushing water was making him want to go to the bathroom. So from then on, I encouraged him to use the bathroom first when he said he was going outside. This helped and after a couple of days it wasn't a problem anymore.

By the end of the week, I was ready for Marilyn to move in. I was ready for anyone to move in. My bookkeeping clients had been very understanding by allowing me to deal with only priority paperwork while Gerry was in the hospital. I had stopped by their offices on my way to the hospital each morning to take what I could. When Gerry was resting, I worked on their books. The rest waited until I got home at night. Now that we were home, I needed some time to get my business reorganized. The other problem was I could only bill clients for the actual hours worked, so my income was reduced accordingly.

Fortunately, Gerry's salary continued to be paid every two weeks. However, there wasn't much left by the time I paid the mortgage, utilities, and groceries. Now the little bit I was earning had to pay Marilyn's salary first so I could bill the RCMP. There were unexpected expenses for Gerry as well, such as shoes. His balance was still unstable. The occupational therapist recommended he have a top quality running shoe because he needed the stability. These were very expensive and not something I had budgeted for.

I tried to do the books with Gerry at home, but it aggravated him. His moods continually shifted from one extreme to the other. In the hospital, he acted as if he couldn't stand to be with me. Now, after only being home a few days, he wanted all my attention. I was like an elastic band ready to snap.

A Change of Mind

Happy Father's Day

It was like old home week the day Marilyn moved in. Myriah and Dale adored Aunty Marilyn. She'd always given freely of her time when visiting. For hours, she'd play the piano for the girls or have tea parties for them. Leaving them in her care was as comfortable as leaving them with their grandmother. Gerry was very fond of her too. She was famous, in his eyes, for her fabulous cooking. Over the years when Marilyn visited, Gerry coerced her into baking homemade buns. No arguments from me!

Marilyn had been a very good friend to me. She was always helpful when she came to visit. Her cooking was out of this world and she never hesitated to pick up a cleaning rag. That's what we needed, someone who would readily pitch in and help. Marilyn's duties also involved caring for Gerry as needed.

It was difficult to know which he needed more, supervision or companionship. He was very childlike in the sense that he had no perception of the consequences of his actions, like going to the bathroom outside. Many times it reminded me of caring for my daughters when they were toddlers, knowing it meant trouble when they were the quietest. He wasn't able to resume his normal activities or hobbies like reading or puttering around in his workshop. Details were simply too frustrating for him. Reading directions or looking at a book held no enjoyment. The letters registered as nothing more than black marks on the sheet of paper.

Gradually his sense of balance was restored and he was able to walk without staggering. He began to enjoy walking so much that it soon became a major part of his day and helped ease his restlessness. Every morning, he and Marilyn set out for a walk and sometimes again in the afternoon.

I was able to resume my bookkeeping business. There was no way I could handle full-time work, so I limited myself to four hours a day outside the house. I scheduled my clients on staggered days so I could go into their offices for the four hours and get caught up on the backlog. What I didn't get done in those four hours simply had to wait for the next day, or until I could squeeze in a few minutes in my office at home.

One thing to look forward to was the school year coming to a close. That was a relief for all of us. I wanted life to be simple again. A couple of months without the rigidity of school bedtimes, making lunches, squeezing in school activities, and doing homework were things we easily could do without on our daily agenda.

Gerry had always loved spending time with our children. Whenever he could help out at school he did. He also took pleasure in taking the girls fishing or hunting for small game, like quail. I thought now having them home all day would be comforting to him. I was depending on his progress accelerating by being with them. The down side was my concern that his need to be with them would be too consuming. Because in many ways he was more childlike than they were, I feared our daughters would be trapped into becoming a parent to him, especially during my absence. Mind you, the kids were great. Not once did they complain about the demands Gerry made on their time.

Not being the father he was prior to the accident was a very big fear for Gerry; so big, he became obsessed with it. We discussed this with the doctors. Unfortunately, Gerry couldn't articulate his fears about parenting. I wasn't much help for the doctors either, because I did not know anything more than that he was depressed.

It was about this time that I succeeded in having Gerry start to keep a journal. I had been keeping a daily journal since the accident to record his moods, appetite, conversation, desires and sleep patterns. The idea behind this was to remind me what I needed to talk to the doctors about. Also, as a police officer's wife, I knew years would pass before his case got into court. I wasn't very confident I would be able to remember the necessary details several years down the road so, for me, keeping a record was the logical thing to do.

Gerry began to question me about writing in the "red book." I explained what I was writing and why. However, he had it stuck in his mind that I was doing this to show the doctors that he needed to be put back in the hospital. The only way I thought I could diffuse his fears was to read my notes to him and encourage him to record his feelings to share with me. Instantly he liked the idea. We went to the office supply store and purchased him a red book, exactly like mine.

At first, the actual mechanics of forming letters were difficult for him. He scrawled big letters across the page and sometimes the sentence was made up of a string of words which made no sense. When he shared these writings, I did my best to decipher them and to refrain from commenting on sentence structure or appearance. He began with the date and, from there, included information about what time he woke up, what he ate, what he did during the day and what time he went to bed.

Gerry began to really enjoy these times with me. I too noticed a transformation in our relationship. The hostility began to subside and I no longer felt as though I were walking around on eggshells. Keeping a journal soon became addictive for him. It was for me too. When Gerry got upset, he couldn't tell me why or even exactly what it was that was bothering him, so I got him to write about his feelings in his journal. There was always hope he'd write some vital information, but this was rare. He did, however, often get himself through a weepy part of the day by writing. Many times these entries led him to a new topic, which was a "gold nugget" because it gave him something to focus on other than how poorly he was feeling.

The month of June was coming to a close. The sunshine increased the temperature a little more each day. Mother Nature always made things better. For me, life always felt manageable if the sun was shining. Besides, the nice weather gave us a reason to be outside. We needed to create some space between us.

Gerry began to putter out in the yard. The key for him was not to take on anything too big or he got frustrated when he couldn't do it. The frustration led to poor self-esteem, which dumped him quickly into a depression. That's what happened on Father's Day.

"Happy Father's Day, Daddy," beamed Dale. Her long dark braids flipped over his shoulder as she hugged him.

"Thanks, Dale," he replied, tears filling his eyes. "God, I love you." He hung onto her. Myriah waited patiently behind her sister. Gerry finally saw her and reached out to include her in the hug.

"Happy Father's Day, Dad," she said, sounding more grownup than her sister did. Her bottom lip quivered as she hugged him. By then, Gerry was sobbing.

I too had to fight back the tears. Everything was so hard for him. His emotions overwhelmed all of us. I jumped in offering our gift as an attempt to lift everyone's spirits.

"Here, Honey. Open your gift. The girls and I thought we could use it for camping or picnics." I placed the heavy package wrapped in Father's Day paper on the table beside him.

Gerry placed a hand on top of the box; his other arm still wrapped around the girls. Stepping back from the table, I sat in the lawn chair beside him, playfully patting his leg. "Come on, Honey. Open it! I know you'll love it."

Seconds later, the ribbon and paper lay in a crinkled heap on the wood deck. The box was opened, revealing little plastic bags with metal pieces, screws, bolts, and knobs. An instruction sheet with diagrams was included, which ultimately was to result in a tabletop propane barbecue.

Dabbling and puttering had always been a passion with Gerry. Like most men, even though he rarely read instructions, he managed to put items together piece by piece. I took it for granted he could do it this time. Apparently, he did too.

I left Gerry basking in the sun to put his gift together and went inside to make lunch. Half an hour later, I stepped onto the deck with a tray of sandwiches, fresh vegetables, and one of Gerry's favorite treats – glazed donuts. Myriah and Dale accompanied me carrying glasses and chilled cans of soda pop. I fully expected to see the barbecue halfway assembled.

Instead, the pieces, big and small, were spread all over the table. Plastic wrappers scattered the deck. Gerry sat with his head tipped back against the outside wall of the house. One hand covered his eyes. The other held the sheet of instructions, trembling.

"Honey, what's wrong?" I asked, putting the tray down on an empty chair.

"I can't do this!" he cried.

"What? What can't you do?"

"This!" His eyes wet with frustration looked pleadingly at the page.

Instantly, I realized my mistake. It was horrible, almost cruel. Gerry couldn't follow the instructions! He couldn't read all the words, and the diagram with lines going in different directions all over the page only confused him. With his abstract thinking so out of whack he couldn't even find where to begin.

I scooped up the parts and bits and threw them into the box as fast as I could. "It's okay, Honey. Let's leave it for a week or two. Then maybe we can figure it out together. Okay?"

"Okay," he mumbled, handing me the tear stained paper.

Two weeks later, Gerry called me outside when I arrived home from work. There he was in the same spot as he had been on Father's Day. This time though, a big grin was splashed across his face. The barbecue was assembled.

"Thanks for making me wait," he said, squeezing me hard. "You were right. It just went together fine today. I don't know why I couldn't do it two weeks ago!"

"The main thing is you did it now, Hon, and it's fine. You can be really pleased with yourself," I told him. Every day he showed some improvement. At times like this, when he was confident and full of self-respect, he seemed like his old self again.

It would have been lovely if every day could have ended as happily as that. But it didn't. More often than not, each day was a roller coaster ride. One day was up, the next was down and you couldn't foresee that an experience would be unhappy one.

On June 28, 1990, Gerry's Aunt Elaine, who was one of the last links to his father's side of the family, arrived from Saskatchewan. Every five years there was a Simon/Breese Family Reunion and this year it was scheduled to be held in Penticton over the long weekend. Our family, including Gerry's brother Dan, was the only family still to retain the "Breese" family name.

When the accident happened, relatives called with concern and also to see if we should postpone the event. Something inside of me said "No," so I insisted it go ahead. Arrangements were in place for out of town guests to stay in one location, a combination motel/campground. Our family and Dan were the only locals, so we opted to stay in our homes. Aunty Elaine was staying with us. It had been several years since we'd seen her. She and her late sister Norma were Gerry's very favorite relatives. I was really excited about her coming to stay. Gerry needed to have his family around him and I was certain he would enjoy seeing everyone at the reunion.

Marilyn went all out helping to get the house in order and a room ready for Elaine. An entire day had been spent baking and stocking the freezer with goodies to enjoy over coffee. Gerry and the girls stayed home with Marilyn when I went to the airport to pick up Elaine. The plane was late by about 30 minutes which put my arrival home nearly an hour behind schedule. Gerry was outside pacing in the gravel driveway when we arrived home. He looked sad and scared. Not the look I expected considering he hadn't seen his aunt in a long, long time.

"Hi, Hon," I said, stepping out of the car. Before Aunty Elaine could get out of the car, Gerry lunged forward, grabbing my arm.

"Where have you been? It's past one o'clock. You scared me." His voice was strained.

"Gerry, you're hurting my arm." My fingers worked to ease his grip. "I'm sorry. The plane was late. We got here as soon as we could."

"Don't do it again. It scares me," he responded, clenching his teeth.

Aunty Elaine was now standing beside us. Gentle lines creased around her eyes as she smiled at her nephew who'd been a breath away from death. Gerry took a bag of groceries from my arms and nonchalantly glanced at his aunt.

"Hi, Aunty Elaine," was all he said as we walked toward the house. I was baffled how he could be so indifferent to someone he adored and hadn't seen in years. Aunty Elaine didn't question, nor did I attempt to discuss it. I was learning his moods could change as quickly as an afternoon rain shower can change into a full-fledged storm.

Two days later all of us headed into town to attend the family reunion. Aunty Elaine and I had shown Gerry family pictures of people

A Change of Mind

who would be attending to help jog his memory. My concern was that he would be as indifferent to them as he had been to his aunt when she arrived. I didn't want them to be offended, nor did I want to offend Gerry by making excuses for him if his reactions weren't appropriate.

The afternoon was hot with no sign of clouds in the sky. The campground was opposite the lake so a few family members were swimming when we arrived. However, many of the relatives were waiting in anticipation.

Gerry clenched the car door handle as we parked. His eyes shifted from left to right, scanning the tourists in the campground and those walking nearby.

"Who are these people?" he asked.

"I don't know, Honey. Just tourists, I guess. Look there are your cousins, Gordon and Ruth!"

Gerry ignored me. He wouldn't let go of the door handle. I got out of the car followed by Aunty Elaine, Myriah and Dale. Both girls hovered at my side as I walked around to the passenger side to open Gerry's door.

"Why isn't Daddy getting out?" asked Dale.

"He's just a little uncertain about remembering names," I reassured her. The sun skipped off the top of her chestnut colored hair as I gently patted her head.

Relatives closed in around the car as I opened the door. Everyone was smiling, anxious to make contact with him. I exchanged greetings as Gerry got out of the car. He gripped my hand, resisting each step as we moved forward. I looked at him, trying to determine his reactions. It took only seconds for arms to clasp around his neck as each one greeted him, expressing words of love and happiness for his survival. Instead of reciprocating with affection, Gerry began to cry. At first, I thought he was just overwhelmed by the outpouring of love. But that didn't seem to be the case. With no explanation he turned away, pulling me towards the car.

"What's the matter, Gerry?

"I don't know!"

"Why are you so upset?" I continued.

"I don't know," he repeated, letting go of my hand so he could open the car door.

Gerry sat in the car with his legs stretched outside. His hands were clenched and tucked between his thighs. He gently rocked back and forth. I knelt in front of him, resting my hands on his legs. I didn't know what to say, because I had no idea what was wrong. Both our daughters stood behind me.

"It's okay, girls. You go sit with Aunty Elaine. I'll stay with Daddy."

"What's the matter?" asked Myriah.

"I think it's just overwhelming for Daddy to see everyone. He hasn't seen them for a long time." My eyes met with the girls. Even at their youthful ages, their expressions suggested they weren't convinced by my explanation. Rising to my feet, I wrapped my arms around them.

"Give Daddy a few minutes. Then we'll come over and sit with everyone. Okay?" I said, adding a tender kiss on each of their heads. Dale kicked her toe to push the gravel beneath her feet away. I gave them each a little pat on the behind, nudging them toward Aunty Elaine, who joyfully took them into the crowd to show them off.

Still rocking, Gerry was crying even harder. I sighed. Should I take him home? Should we wait it out? It would probably embarrass him if I said we were leaving. Instinct told me we'd regret it if we did.

The solution was to wait it out as it had been so many times in the past few weeks. He and I stayed at the car for nearly 45 minutes. Slowly his mood settled and he regained composure. Finally, he made the choice to get out of the car and go sit with his family. For weeks, Gerry told me over and over how glad he was that I didn't just whisk him away that day. Sticking it out and participating in the family reunion for the entire weekend gave Gerry renewed strength and a sense of wholeness.

This new courage allowed him to start taking more control of his life by trying new things. One of the lagging problems, however, was his inability to perceive consequences for his actions. This became very obvious when I took him driving for the first time.

Driving had been a part of his life since age 13, when he drove on his family's farm. Also, being a police officer meant Gerry had to meet the requirements of defensive driving. He specialized in traffic and was capable of driving at high speeds. He could tell you within a small margin what speed a car was traveling just by sight.

I was against Gerry getting behind the wheel of a car so soon. It soon became a constant argument. He didn't seem ready to me. It had only been seven weeks since the accident. But he persisted and I agreed to go with the doctors' decision. So we made appointments. Since there were three professionals involved (our family physician, a neurologist and a neuropsychologist), I felt confident in having at least a 2-1 decision against Gerry driving.

The first doctor felt very confident in Gerry's ability to begin driving. "Driving is something you never forget," he said. "Much like a bicycle." I explained I didn't feel Gerry had forgotten the techniques. I felt he wasn't able to cope with all the activity such as controlling speed while simultaneously reading street signs, watching for children on the road and obeying traffic control signals. The doctor's decision remained a yes vote. Gerry was ecstatic. As far as he was concerned there was no need to seek further advice.

At my insistence, we proceeded to the second appointment. This doctor voted no. In his opinion Gerry wasn't ready to handle an activity as abstract as driving. This plummeted Gerry to a deep low. It was now at his insistence that we obtain a third opinion as a tiebreaker.

Taking time to thoroughly explain to the third doctor Gerry's abilities and reactions to various activities, I hoped he'd side with the doctor who voted no. However, at the end of my long explanation he looked at us and simply said, "Well, maybe."

As hard as I tried to get a firm decision from this man, positive or negative, he sat on the fence. Gerry burst into tears right in this doctor's office, because he too had hoped for a tiebreaker. Gerry's emotional outburst should have been a sign he wasn't ready for a highly stressful and responsible activity like driving.

We left the office, both of us disappointed in the outcome. Regardless of the fact that each of us hoped for an opposite answer, the bottom line was we needed a professional to help us make a decision. We felt let down. It would have saved a tremendous amount of heartache and frustration if Gerry could have taken a driving test to determine his abilities. To the best of my knowledge, no such test existed then.

Gerry kept up the pressure for a day or two, and finally I decided to let him drive our small Toyota to the village store with me supervising from the passenger side. It was what I should have done in the beginning. Gerry drove the car out of the driveway without looking in either direction for oncoming traffic. Fortunately, there wasn't any. He continued down the road, a steady decline, into the lower part of the village. His foot pressed heavy on the gas pedal. I panicked.

"Gerry, slow down. You're going too fast!"

"No, I'm not."

"Yes, you are. Do you know what the speed limit is?" I asked.

"Speed limit?" he replied. "You just drive as fast as you know how. That's all."

His answers confirmed my fears. He had not forgotten how to drive, but he was a hazard on the road! On the drive back home, it was the more of the same. We argued about speed. My heart nearly stopped when he didn't see an elderly woman run out to the road to retrieve her little poodle who was headed directly into our path.

My nerves were frazzled as the Toyota lurched to a stop in the gravel driveway. Gerry took the keys out of the ignition. I quickly scooped them from his hand, telling him he wasn't ready to drive. I'd like to be able to say he understood, but he didn't. He was furious.

Ironically, several weeks later when Gerry was out for a drive with our friend, Maurice Tremblay, the purpose of a posted speed limit became clear to him. Gerry noticed the traffic sign that said 30 km/h. As Maurice slowed the vehicle down, Gerry realized what was happening and said, "Hey. I just figured out what Janelle meant. When a sign says 30 kilometers an hour, it means to slow the car down to 30 kilometers." That revelation was tremendous progress for all of us. Soon after this incident, Gerry was able to drive short distances. He was still very fatigued during the day and needed several naps, which made me leery about letting him drive anywhere for more than a few minutes at a time.

Once the hurdle of driving was over, Gerry couldn't understand why the rest of his life was not back to normal. For him this was about his inability to return to work. For me, it was about our inability as a family to return to the way we were prior to the accident. Our lives had changed dramatically. Absolutely nothing had remained the same. Each and every one of us had been transformed by the experience, including our children.

Gerry and I were not your "Barbie and Ken" couple. We were just an average husband and wife who loved being parents to our daughters and thrived on our family and community involvements. Our marriage was strong, yet over the years it had been subjected to the typical ups and downs that most couples experience. It had even survived gouges so deep that traces of irreparable scars lingered such as the devastating murder of his younger brother by a family friend and Gerry's extramarital affair as we approached our sixth wedding anniversary. As painful as those experiences were, and certainly ones that I never wanted to go through again, we were able to overcome the desolation and see our love strengthened in spite of the experience. Although these tumultuous times transformed us in some way, the essence of who we were individually and as a couple remained the same. But since Gerry's brain injury, he wasn't remotely close to being the man I married. He was a complete stranger to me.

In a matter of weeks our relationship as lovers and friends had been altered – physically and emotionally. Now when Gerry reached for my hand or I reached for his, it was to convey his need to feel safe or it was my response to calm his fears rather than the loving or even sensual communication that it had been before.

There was no longer any flirting or sexual banter between us either. Our conversations were strictly about soothing him, about medical or legal appointments, about his fears, his frustrations, and what it was going to take to get him through the day. Period. All the other details which we previously shared, like parenting, planning our day, week or month, work, fun … anything at all… were left up to me to handle.

And if I couldn't cope with it on my own, our daughters had to step up to the plate and assist me. And if it was something our children couldn't cope with, then I had to turn to family and friends. However, there is only so much that children, family and friends can do for you. They could not fill the void I was feeling as a woman and a wife. This was a path I had to walk alone. Nonetheless, it didn't stop the professionals from assuming that our intimacy had remained intact. For example, shortly after Gerry was home we had a visit from his occupational therapist. She spent some time with Gerry alone and then asked to speak privately with me. As we sat sipping our coffee, she inquired about how life was between us as husband and wife.

"So if you don't mind me asking, how is your sex life? Everything back to normal?" she asked.

"Pardon me?" I asked, truly astonished.

"Your sex life - have you and Gerry been able to resume your sex life?"

"Isn't that a little incestuous?" I asked sarcastically. It was now she who was astonished.

"Why do you say incestuous?"

"Because he is like a little boy!" I blurted, feeling quite frustrated that no one but me seemed to see that our relationship had changed. Furthermore, I was physically and emotionally exhausted. Having sex was the furthest thing from my mind.

To her credit, this woman was completely changed by our conversation. She told me that from that day forward she never ever made the assumption again that a husband and wife would, or could, just pick up where they left off prior to one of them sustaining a brain injury.

For Gerry, he went from being quite aggressive sexually to not being interested at all in those few weeks. He was much more concerned with what other people were thinking about him not returning to work.

It was now nearing the end of July and all his physical injuries had pretty much healed. He looked great. Physically that is. Instead of being happy about this, Gerry started to get paranoid and feared his co-workers thought him nothing more than a fake.

A Change of Mind

"They don't believe that I'm sick any more," he would say after a visit from people he worked with. "They think I'm just faking. They think that I can go back to work because I don't have stitches anymore or a cast."

Right about this time Gerry had a scheduled visit with Dr. Novak. He could see the stress not being able to return to work caused Gerry. As at previous appointments, Gerry cried uncontrollably. He believed he was letting down the officers he worked with.

Dr. Novak and I had a lengthy discussion behind closed doors about this. Our best guess was that part of the problem was the approaching August long weekend. The sunshine and sandy beaches in Penticton beckon partygoers to come and enjoy extended weekends. This presents a very severe strain on the Penticton detachment and hundreds of officers are recruited throughout the province to help out. This was the first year in five that Gerry wasn't scheduled to work on that weekend. Nobody was ever given that weekend off. This stuck in his mind. Inspector Thompsett, John Turnell, Curtis Horton, and Hughie Winters tried to assure him they knew he would go back to work if he could. Nothing eased the pain for him.

Dr. Novak recommended we go out of town for a while, especially over that weekend. It was a perfect solution! We had just purchased a newer Oldsmobile and I felt secure enough to take the month of August and travel.

The first stop would be to visit my sister Rachel and her husband Bob. Their three children, Joshua, Desmond and Anthony, always enjoyed getting together with Myriah and Dale. From there I planned to drive to McBride, B.C., which is situated between the northern city of Prince George and the Alberta border, to visit our friends Nelson and Bobbie-Ann Hicks. It had been fifteen years since Gerry had seen Nelson. However, Nelson had read about Gerry's accident in the Vancouver newspaper and came to visit him in the Kelowna hospital. I was astonished that Gerry recognized Nelson when he walked into his hospital room. Immediately, Gerry referred to Nelson by his high school nickname "Crash". Those early days were pretty much a blur for Gerry and he did not remember Nelson coming to visit. After McBride we were going to Peace River, Alberta to visit Natalie and her family, Dave, Ben and Katie.

For three days I studied maps and worked out our itinerary. It was a long way to go. It would take three and a half weeks to complete the trip. But I knew that seeing our relatives and close friends would be a warming boost for Gerry. We needed this time as a family. It didn't matter that we would be in the car for eight hours a day. The fact was we would be spending time together. Just the four of us.

The night before leaving, we made a special point of going to visit Bob and Ruth. It had been a while since I had seen Ruth and I couldn't help feeling something was very different about her. It wasn't what she said. It was more of a physical change, especially her face and eyes.

Bob and Gerry chatted about the office. I sat quietly while Ruth cleaned out a purse, not acknowledging our presence. This was highly unusual, because Ruth and I could talk for hours whenever we got together. Tonight she seemed indifferent to me. She hadn't been feeling well since May and was experiencing increasingly more seizures.

When we said goodbye that evening, I hugged her. She reminded me of our upcoming plans together. "Don't forget. We're all going to the brain injury conference in October. Bob booked the time off and we can drive down together."

"Oh, I won't forget. Our registration has been in for a while. I'm looking forward to it." Ruth was talking about the Pacific Coast Brain Injury Conference being held in Vancouver in mid October. This annual event brings together survivors of brain injury, their families and friends, professionals and caregivers. The goals are to increase the understanding of problems faced by survivors and their families, as well as to introduce the current services available and future programs. Okanagan Rehabilitation and Consulting Ltd. in Kelowna had provided Ruth with the information for registration. She had not wanted to go, but she agreed to attend after Gerry's accident when I said we would go with her and Bob.

"How about Gerry? Is he looking forward to going too?" she asked.

"Well, I'm not sure, but I'm certain he'll be okay once we go."

"Yeah. We'll have great fun." Ruth waved goodbye to us as we walked to the car. My eyes met hers when I glanced back one last time. Something was so wrong.

A Family Vacation

The brilliant morning sun heated the car windows as we headed north on the highway, leaving all our worries and concerns behind in Penticton.

Myriah and Dale giggled in the back seat as they planned out their road trip activities. Piled on the seat between them were their favorite books, paper, crayons, and stuffed toys.

Gerry relaxed in the passenger seat, gazing across the lake listening to me talk. I was explaining the changes I planned to make on our return home. Changes I hoped he approved of.

Prior to leaving on holidays, Gerry and I had met with our lawyer Gordon Marshall. He was prepared to oversee our court action but had asked his colleague Robin Adolphe, who had previous experience with brain injury claims, to be in charge of the case. Immediately, Robin contacted John Simpson of Simpson Rehabilitation in Vancouver, whose company coordinates available services for families and survivors. John met with us and suggested we work with Christine Lefaivre, the founder of Okanagan Rehabilitation and Consulting Ltd., who was closer to home.

We were familiar with Chris, because she had worked with Ruth since her accident. Both Ruth and Bob raved about the support and care her company provided their family.

From the moment Gerry and I met Chris, we liked and trusted her. After hearing her personal story of a spinal injury as a teenager, I understood clearly why her success rate with clients was so high. She had first hand experience with the frustrations and setbacks that could occur during recovery. Chris appreciated the feelings of exhilaration that accompanied small victories. She knew how to make them happen!

Chris' success with families and survivors of brain injury stems from her treatment of the body, mind and spirit together. Healing one without the others is impractical and incongruent.

In our meetings with Chris, I discussed Gerry's lingering depression. Taking into consideration his lifestyle as a police officer before the accident, Chris and I wondered if part of the problem was a lack of male companionship. His days were now spent with our daughters, Marilyn, and me.

Chris suggested we take steps to restore our family unit and his self-esteem by replacing Marilyn with a male caregiver. The decision was no reflection on the care Marilyn had given. Her work was impeccable and her love shone through everything she did. It was simply an option we had to explore. I agreed to have Chris find a suitable replacement. This time, however, the caregiver would work on a Monday to Friday, 9-5 basis. We would spend the evenings and weekends by ourselves as we had done in the past. These treasured times were always relaxing and low key. In a typical evening, we would sit around in our housecoats and watch television or play games with the girls. On the weekends, we would putter around the house or go shopping. At least once over the weekend we would get together with my family for lunch or dinner.

Gerry was going to miss having Marilyn around, but he understood the idea behind the change and agreed to it. He was excited about having a man to talk with, someone he could go fishing with or just be with him to dilly-dally around the house. For me, it meant that I could get the girls ready to go back to school and establish a regular workweek for myself when we returned from holidays at the end of August.

Taking this vacation was the first step in resuming activities as a family. It had required a little creative planning on my part to get Gerry to agree to go away. He liked the idea of going to visit everyone, but he was very fearful of leaving family in Penticton – especially my brother Nathan. To ease his concerns, Nathan and his family decided to travel with us for the first leg of our trip to William's Lake where we would visit with our sister Rachel. She and I had planned a mini family reunion for the weekend. After that we would continue on our trip to Peace River and Nathan and his family would return home.

Our first night at Rachel's set the tone for the duration of our holiday. The benefits were obvious. Gerry needed to get his feelings out. The only way to do that was to talk about the accident and his recovery. This wasn't easy for him. One had to be very careful to listen, encouraging him to keep dealing with his feelings as he got them out.

Having new faces and fresh ears to hear his story was helpful. They could listen intently because it was the first time they had heard his story. But they also offered enthusiastic support and suggestions. I have to admit, my energy to do that had dwindled over the months.

Along with the benefits there were, of course, drawbacks – drawbacks that could not have been foreseen. They were simply a result of his everchanging moods and discoveries.

One instance in particular stands out. Gerry had a bad dream the first night we were at Rachel's. Myriah, who was only 12 years old at the time, appeared in the dream as though she were 18. She was getting married and naturally expected her father would escort her down the aisle to give her away. Myriah's fiancé was embarrassed at her father's obvious deficits. After her future husband complained, someone in the dream told Myriah she couldn't have her "brain-dead" father give her away.

Gerry woke up from the dream crying. He kept saying he felt so ashamed. Ashamed the accident had happened. Ashamed for putting his family through this difficult and trying time. Ashamed he wasn't back at work and that he might never be able to return to work again. Most of all, he felt ashamed of not being capable of doing the fatherly things he had done for his children prior to the accident. These chains were of his own making. Nothing we said or did eased his pain. It was something he had to work through on his own.

After we left Rachel's house, we took our time traveling to Peace River. We did all the typical tourist things. We ate our meals out, shopped and took in the attractions. Some were new. Some, like the waterslide, were just family favorites.

Many happy hours had been spent as a family at the Penticton waterslide, so I was thrilled when we got to Natalie's and discovered there was an indoor slide at the community center. The girls couldn't wait to go. We quickly cemented plans to go the next afternoon.

I offered to take my three year old nephew Ben, and one year old niece Katie with us. There was a small wading pool that I was certain they would enjoy.

After arriving at the community center, I directed Gerry toward the men's changing room. The four children came with me into the women's room. Echoes of splashing and laughter filled the room where we took turns stepping under the tepid showers. Myriah and Dale received my final instructions on the rules of water safety before we all proceeded, hand in hand, to the pool area. Humidity and the stench of chlorine filled our lungs as we crossed the threshold from the showers to the indoor playland.

When we turned the corner, I could see Gerry standing against the cement wall with his arms folded over his chest. His body was trembling and he stared at me with wide fear-filled eyes. A funny sensation whirled in the pit of my stomach. "What's the matter, Gerry?" I asked, rushing to his side.

"I'm scared!" His eyes glazed over. His deep voice cracked.

"Scared of what?"

"I don't know."

I slipped my arm through his while balancing Katie on one hip and keeping an eye on Ben. Myriah and Dale scurried past us.

"We're going down the waterslide, Mom. See ya!"

I gave a quick nod as they disappeared. Ben pulled my hand, wanting to get into the wading pool.

"Come on, Gerry. Let's get in the pool with Ben and Katie," I encouraged.

"I can't!" he replied, planting his feet firmly on the cement patio.

"You can't?" I asked. "Why?"

"I'm scared, Janelle. I'm scared."

A young woman with a small girl slowed down as they walked by. The woman glanced over her shoulder at Gerry. An elderly man and woman, sitting on white plastic patio chairs, stared in our direction. I wanted to scream at them – all of them.

I could not understand Gerry's sudden fear of water. He had his bronze medallion in swimming from the RCMP. I couldn't disappoint the kids by not staying, so I pleaded with him to sit in the shallowest part of the wading pool with Ben and Katie and me.

The water was only ankle deep and it barely covered our thighs when we were sitting. Katie sat between my legs splashing happily as babies do. Ben was content beside me with a slew of small toys. Gerry was on the opposite side of me, his hands holding tightly to my upper arm.

Eventually his grip loosened and he actually began to enjoy himself. When he realized how much fun he was having, watching the girls come down the slide, he was elated with his achievement. Overcoming obstacles like this became major victories for Gerry. He was overjoyed once he faced and confronted his fears.

We spent nearly a week with Natalie and her family before beginning our journey home. I had planned to take about six days to get back to Penticton. Four of those days were going to be spent in Wells, B.C., a small mining town ninety miles east of Quesnel where our good friends Maurice and Sandee Tremblay lived. Gerry, Maurice and Bob Ogden had worked together on the same shift in Penticton prior to Maurice's transfer and Gerry's accident. For Gerry, this was going to one of the highlights. He was really looking forward to spending time with Maurice, who not only was one of his best friends, but also a police officer.

The first three days were spent catching up and exploring the town with Maurice and Sandee. Gerry even went into the small detachment office with Maurice for a while one day. The rest of the time seemed like pure indulgence – we laughed, we ate, and we talked. For the first time since May, I felt as though our family was whole.

The night before we were to go home, Maurice was on call. I hadn't heard the phone ring at seven o'clock that morning. When we got up, Maurice told us he had gone to the office but didn't elaborate. Nor did we ask. It wasn't important. So I thought.

I had finished packing our suitcases and went into the living room with a cup of coffee. Sandee was getting dressed. Gerry was outside watching Myriah and Dale play ball. Maurice was seated on the couch with his legs outstretched and crossed. He looked very upset. I wondered if it had anything to do with Gerry, but I was afraid to ask.

A few minutes of silence weighed heavily in the room. Finally Maurice spoke. He didn't move a muscle. The words came softly.

"Bob called this morning. That's why I went to the office."

"Bob … Bob Ogden? " I asked. My heart skipped a beat. Something was wrong! "What's happened, Maurice? Is it Ruth?" My mouth was dry. No matter how hard I tried to swallow, I couldn't.

Maurice turned his head slightly to look at me. "Yeah, it's Ruth. It looks bad."

My eyelids slowly shut. I wasn't certain I wanted to hear any more. Maurice quietly explained his conversation with Bob. They had received the results from tests that Ruth had done before we left on holidays. There was no doubt. Ruth had an inoperable brain tumor. The doctors expected that she would live only a couple of months at best.

"Have you told Sandee?" I queried, resting my hand on his shoulder.

"No, I haven't. I wanted to tell you first, so we could tell Sandee and Gerry together." His dark eyes were moist with the reality of this painful news. I breathed deeply. It would be difficult to find the right words to tell Gerry. Sandee unexpectedly came into the room. There was no way to hide our feelings.

Maurice explained to Sandee what the early morning telephone call had been about. She crumbled. He took Sandee in his arms to console her. I left the room.

The screen door was propped open. Gerry and the girls were putting the suitcases into the trunk. My heart pounded. How could I tell him about Ruth? She was his lifeline. As long as Ruth was getting better, Gerry believed he would too. I did not want this news to make him give up hope.

Gerry slammed the lid of the trunk closed, turning to see me in the doorway. "Hi. You ready to go?" He took each of the girls by the hand.

"I think you should come in for a minute. There is something we need to talk about. How about you girls playing outside for a few more minutes while Dad and I talk?"

The girls let go of their Dad's hand, and ran toward the ball they had left on the grass. Gerry followed me into Sandee and Maurice's trailer. Sobs could be heard from the living room. Gerry looked frightened as he followed the muffled sound. We went into the living room where Sandee was still cradled in Maurice's arms.

"Something has happened, hasn't it?"

"Sit down and let me explain," I replied, taking his hand and guiding him to the armchair. Kneeling in front of him, I clasped both my hands over his. Slowly and steadily I told him of Ruth's prognosis. I tried to keep my eyes on his, but the pain he felt was unbearable to see. He lurched his body back in the chair, wailing with anger at the injustice of her illness.

"No! No! She doesn't deserve this!" he shouted.

It did not take long for Myriah and Dale to hear the shouting and come inside to satisfy their youthful curiosity. There was no point withholding the news from them. Both girls were quite the troopers and I had long ago come to the conclusion that honesty was the best way with them. With the compassion of an adult, these two little girls moved quickly to wrap their arms around each other and then around their Dad.

By then, everyone was crying – everyone but me, that is. I was numb. I was angry. I was in total disbelief. Discreetly, I got up and disappeared into the bedroom to phone Bob. His voice sounded weary when he answered the telephone. All I said was "Hello" and he fell apart. I knew Maurice's facts were accurate, but I needed to hear it myself. It took only two words from Bob for the reality to sink in.

"Ruth's dying," he said. The words echoed mournfully over the telephone. The few hundred miles between us may as well have been thousands. I wanted to be with them, to hold them, to tell them how sorry we were. The Ogdens had been our closest friends in Penticton, an absolute fortress of strength these past few months. It would be unthinkable to not reciprocate in their time of need.

Words rambled from my mouth. We would leave for home immediately. I told Bob, knowing it would be a grueling 14 hour trip. It didn't matter. I wanted to see Ruth. He assured me Ruth wanted to see me and asked me to come and visit her in the morning.

Sandee decided to come home with us. Her parents live in Penticton, so she could spend a few days with them making it a mini holiday for herself. She could also help with the driving.

Within the hour, Sandee, Gerry, the kids and I said our goodbyes to Maurice and headed out for the long trip south.

There was not much of the night left when we pulled ourselves into bed. It wouldn't have made any difference if there had been. We didn't sleep for long, or peacefully. Ruth was on my mind the entire time. Long before it was an appropriate hour to make telephone calls or go visiting, Gerry and I were up sipping coffee.

Around 10:00 a.m. I received a telephone call from Hugh and Patti Winters. As tactfully as she could, Patti informed me Ruth didn't want to see anyone. Not even me. Words of sympathy, understanding, and encouragement not to take it personally passed through the phone line. They stung deep. Ruth and I were best friends. We had been through so much together. Besides, just yesterday, Bob told me I could see Ruth today.

"Ruth needs some time," Patti said. "Her parents are here and they have all decided to fly back to Ontario so Ruth can visit the rest of her family."

My voice quivered. Rage bubbled within. I didn't know whom I was angry with. Was I angry with Patti for telling me that Ruth didn't want to see me? Or was I angry with Ruth for not wanting to see me? Or was I just angry at life in general? The tumor was growing, consuming Ruth's life minute by minute, like a monster we couldn't predict or control.

I was really confused over the next four days. Every opportunity I had without Gerry or the kids nearby, I dialed Ruth's telephone number. No one answered. The Ogdens had obviously gone to Ontario. The situation seemed unfair and it hurt.

Over the next few days, I bumped into friends who worked with Bob and Gerry. They knew Ruth and I were close friends and they were naturally concerned. I avoided the subject, because my feelings were so close to the surface.

At the end of the week, Gerry and I had taken the girls out to dinner. After eating, we drove along the lake, stopping to take a few minutes to walk along the shore. The kids looked for small shells, skipping a few stones along the water's surface. The water was so calm it was like a mirror. A sense of peacefulness enveloped me. I didn't want to leave, but soon one of the girls needed a restroom so we headed home.

When I stopped the car in front of our house, I could see cream colored notepaper stuck between the door and its frame. My heart lifted as I read the note. Ruth was home. She wanted to see me. I couldn't get to the telephone fast enough.

Half an hour later we were sitting in the Ogden's family room enjoying a cup of coffee. Ruth talked about their trip and how wonderful it had been to see her sisters. She went on and on about the Blue Jays game they saw. Bob chatted with Gerry while the girls played quietly.

Nothing was said about Ruth's brain tumor. Ruth was far more interested in Gerry's recovery. She was thrilled his appetite was increasing and that he was able to barbecue a meal for us without supervision. She understood how good it felt to regain some control over your life. Even the small things felt good.

I noticed Ruth had forgotten things that I had explained to her before we went away. "How's Marilyn working out?" Ruth asked, obviously forgetting we let Marilyn go.

"Fine. I haven't heard from her for a while," I explained. "Do you remember that I told you there was going to be a man working with Gerry instead of Marilyn?"

"No, I didn't know," Ruth said. She picked up a tea towel and began polishing her purse. I was puzzled. When I looked at Bob he shook his head, mouthing the words to indicate Ruth was having memory lapses.

On September 28th, Ruth was admitted to the hospital. It was Bob's birthday. My birthday is September 30th. Traditionally, we celebrated together. Ruth had not even realized it was Bob's birthday when he took her to the hospital.

Gerry and I and the girls came into town to have dinner with Bob and his girls anyway. Dinner was quiet. We tried to laugh and carry on as we had in times past, but it was hard without Ruth. We already missed her.

The doctor told Bob that the time Ruth had left was perhaps as little as several weeks. In my heart I feared it would be only days. I think Bob did too.

Goodbye to a Friend

It wasn't long before my concern over Ruth's deterioration turned into an obsession – every minute of every hour.

Most days, I went to the hospital to visit Ruth late afternoon around the dinner hour. Bob was often home at that time checking on Heather and Becky. Ruth was usually alone.

Everyone wanted to find some way to help Bob and the girls. By taking a shift at the hospital so he could spend time with the girls, I felt that at least I was contributing. However, it just didn't feel like enough.

At first, these private visits gave Ruth and me some opportunities for long heart-to-heart talks. But after awhile, her motor skills began to decline and even eating her food without assistance was next to impossible. It was heartbreaking for me to see her like that and I'm certain it was devastating for Bob, Heather and Becky as well. So by going to visit her at dinner time, I could at least help her eat.

No matter how limiting her communication ability became, Ruth always recognized me. When she was still able to talk, she always asked about Gerry. Whenever a nurse came into the room, Ruth gave her the full story of how we had met and all that we had been through together. In what seemed like only a matter of days, our visits went from full fledged conversations to a mere word or two. I talked while helping Ruth eat. She listened and occasionally made a sound as though she was trying to say something.

Within a couple of weeks of being hospitalized, I noticed a tremendous difference in Ruth. The glint in her eyes was now gone. Instead, she looked around the room in a dream-like state as I talked. Her frail body was now molded into a piece of sheepskin in an oversized recliner. I just sat with her, not feeling any need to talk. It was good to just be together. There didn't seem to be a need for us to talk. I think we had said it all on a hot afternoon shortly after Ruth was hospitalized.

On that afternoon, I could sense Ruth was withdrawn and sullen when I entered her room. Her head rested against the back of the reclining chair and looked as though it were too heavy for her to move.

Her beautifully rich brown eyes, once filled with an impish sparkle, were now flat and defeated. Ruth bit down on her bottom lip. Her bony hands gripped the arms of the chair.

"Promise me, Janelle. Promise you will always be there for Bob and the girls. Please?" she asked, tears trickling down her freckled cheek. My tears flowed spontaneously.

"I promise Ruth. I'll do whatever I can to help them. Gerry will too. I promise," I said, pulling my chair closer to her and taking her hand.

"I'm so scared," she sobbed. "I'm just so scared." There was nothing I could say to comfort her. I could only imagine how terrified I would be if it were me.

"Ruth, I have to tell you something. I wanted to tell you this for months, but there never seemed to be a good time." My fingers gently massaged her gold wedding band which was now too large for her. "You have been a wonderful friend," I continued. "You have taught me so much. You taught me about friendship. You taught me about facing fear and you taught me about dignity." Ruth moaned softly, her eyes locked onto mine.

The heavy door of her room pushed open. A nurse was coming in for a routine check. Neither Ruth nor I really acknowledged her presence until the nurse asked, "You must be Janelle?" I nodded.

"I've heard so much about you." I smiled.

"Ruth and I are very close," I replied.

"I can see that." The nurse hesitated for a moment and then said, "Ruth needs to let her feelings out. I'm happy she can do it with you."

Ruth and I squeezed each other's hand. Ironically, as best as I can remember this was the last real conversation we had. After that, she communicated only by eye contact. Soon she could no longer even squeeze my hand.

The time had finally come when I knew it was physically and emotionally impossible for me to keep going to the hospital to see her. It was traumatic for Gerry to be left at home. He was having a difficult time understanding how or why Ruth's health was deteriorating so quickly.

A Change of Mind

He was afraid to visit her in the hospital and I didn't think it was in his best interest for him to see her. Each time I came back from visiting her, Gerry cried and cried because he felt so insecure without me at his side.

His grief and my sadness over Ruth began to wear on me. I was physically and emotionally exhausted. I couldn't seem to rejuvenate myself. The bottom line was that if I were to get sick or, to be honest, collapse with a nervous breakdown, it would do none of us any good. So I made the painful decision to say a final goodbye to Ruth.

I was relieved to find no one in Ruth's room when I arrived at the hospital. She wasn't in her chair as I had expected. Her small frame lay beneath a draped sheet on the bed. Her room was cool and filled with shadows. Ruth's back faced the doorway. I tiptoed into the room and around the bed. To my surprise, she was awake. My fingers slipped under her hand.

"Hi, you're not asleep," I said. Ruth's eyes moved to connect with mine, but she didn't speak. She couldn't. "You're not in your chair. I guess it's getting too uncomfortable." Silence filled the room. My throat tightened. There was no point in stalling by making small talk. My voice lowered as I began to speak again.

"Ruth … I know this is hard for you and I know you're scared. And I know you really need your friends and family right now. But I have to be honest with you. I don't think I can be of much help to you right now. It's so difficult for Gerry. He gets very upset when I'm not at home."

I stood quietly. Our eyes were fixed on one another. I reached out to stroke Ruth's head, leaning closer to whisper in her ear. This was going to be hard.

"You have been a wonderful friend, Ruth. Just the best. I'll never forget what you have done for me. I'll never forget the support you and Bob gave Gerry and me and our girls after his accident." My voice cracked and tears streamed down my face. "Ruth … I … I just can't come back any more. I want to be here with you, but Gerry needs me so much right now. I'm sorry. But it's time for me to say goodbye." Those final words poured out in a sob. "I love you, Ruth. I always will. I know we'll meet again." I kissed her cheek. A single tear pooling in the corner of her eye reflected her feelings.

Releasing her hand, I slowly backed away and turned to leave. In my heart, I believed this would be the last time I would see Ruth. And it was. Ruth died peacefully one week later in the early morning of October 15th, 1990.

It just happened that Myriah and Dale had not gone to school that day because the television show *McGyver* was filming where we lived in the village of Naramata. We had been down at the set since 5:30 a.m. waiting for a small glimpse of the star, Richard Dean.

Around 9:30 we went home. I heard the telephone ringing in the kitchen as I hurried to unlock the door. The woman on the other end identified herself as the high school counselor. She asked me to come and get Heather and then told me of Ruth's death. It took a few minutes for the news to sink in so I could tell Gerry and the girls what the call was about. I was amazed at Gerry's response to the news. He barely reacted.

"Where is Bob?" was all he asked. I had no idea. Why had Bob not gone to get Heather himself? Why did he not call me? Later the counselor told me it was Heather who asked her to call me.

Within 35 minutes, Gerry, Myriah, Dale and I had picked Heather up at the school and were on our way to her house. Gerry sat next to me in the front of the car. He said hello to Heather, but nothing more.

Bob met us at the door when we arrived. He held Heather in his arms, letting her cry. One by one we made it through the line to Bob, doing the same as Heather. Everyone except Gerry, that is. He wrapped his arms around Bob's shoulders and simply said, "I'm sorry." Then he went inside to find the kids.

I found Becky, the youngest Ogden girl, huddled on the sofa in the family room, her large brown eyes fixed on the carpet in front of her. God, how she looked like her mother. There were no words to soothe her deep wounds. A hug was all I could muster. I didn't want to interfere with her healing by inflicting my own pain on her. Thank God for children. Myriah and Dale soon had Heather and Becky's minds on other things, which offered them temporary relief from the reality that their mother was never coming home.

Bob was busy taking phone calls and beginning to make arrangements for Ruth's funeral. Gerry helped me clean up and begin preparing food in the kitchen for the arrival of Ruth's family from Ontario. I didn't know what else to do.

Bob was in shock, but at the same time he was very concerned about Gerry. He knew that Ruth's death would be quite upsetting for Gerry. At first, he hesitated to ask Gerry to be a pallbearer. Finally he decided to give him the opportunity. Gerry was deeply moved, vowing to do the best he could.

Ruth's funeral was scheduled for the same day Gerry and I had planned to drive to the Pacific Coast Brain Injury Conference in Vancouver. Ironically, this was the same conference the four of us had planned to attend together. I booked a flight for both of us leaving late Thursday afternoon and returning to Penticton on Sunday night. This way we could attend Ruth's funeral and still make it to the conference. I was certain that Ruth would not have wanted us to miss it.

Gerry looked strikingly handsome in a pale blue suit the day of Ruth's funeral. He had lost quite a bit of weight, making him look so much younger. I was surprised how relaxed he seemed. All morning I had been asking if he wanted to change his mind. He said he didn't.

Myriah and Dale looked pretty. Their long hair glistened in the light. Ruth always described them as "the girls with the long, long braids." I was so proud of the support they had given Heather and Becky.

The pews in the big blue United Church were filled to capacity with police officers, their wives, children and Heather and Becky's many, many school friends.

When we arrived at the church, I took Gerry over to the other pallbearers. Then the girls and I found seating with my Mom and sister. I could easily keep an eye on Gerry from where I was sitting.

It took only a few minutes for Gerry to begin pacing. That wasn't a good sign. He paced and paced. Back and forth. Suddenly, he saw me and darted to the back of the church where I was seated. He began to cry.

"I need a pill. Look at me - I'm shaking," he said, holding his hand horizontally in front of my face. The pill he referred to was Ativan, a nonaddictive relaxant prescribed to relieve anxiety attacks.

"You don't have to do this, Gerry. If you want, I'll ask Bob to get a replacement." I brushed my hand over the material of his suit.

"No! I want to do it for Ruth. I just need a pill to calm me down." I handed him the tiny blue savior. He popped it under his tongue and walked away, taking his place at the front of the church near Ruth's flower draped casket. I studied his every move. I only hoped he would make it through the service.

Unexpectedly, as I watched Gerry resume his pacing, I felt the intense warmth from a hand resting on the back of my neck. Another arm with jangling gold bracelets wrapped around my shoulders and over my chest. The warmth blanketed my ear, as a voice whispered, "How you doing, kid? This must be hard for you." It was Mary MacDonald. Her husband, Jack, was a Staff Sergeant. There was no way I could turn to look at her. I felt a lump swelling in my throat. Soon, I gave way to a floodgate of tears.

My mother tucked tissues into my hand. Two police officers' wives - Alida Erickson and Yvonne Wild - were seated in front of me and turned around and reached over to pat my hand. Everyone sensed how much I'd miss her. All the pain and sorrow I'd tucked away since her death raged forth like a storm out of control. I couldn't stop. I didn't want to stop. I just wanted her back.

Goodbye My Love

Our plane taxied into the Vancouver terminal later that evening. My sister Debby and her husband John had invited us to stay with them. Thankfully they were waiting at the airport to greet us when we arrived. All the noise and large groups of people were unsettling for Gerry. Besides it had been an incredibly long and emotional day.

The next morning, Gerry and I made our way by public transit to the hotel in downtown Vancouver where the Pacific Coast Brain Injury Conference was being held. The weather was typical for Vancouver with a fine mist hovering in the dawn hours that felt cool against my skin. Gerry was very apprehensive about attending the conference. He didn't relish the idea of meeting new people. I had no more idea than he did as to what or whom we would encounter on this adventure, but I was going with an open mind. I was filled with the anticipation of learning about the recoveries of survivors with brain injuries and how their families coped.

I gathered information sheets and a package for each of us at the registration table. It contained a program for the three days with details of each workshop and the intended audience. Many were about survivors and their families, but some were just for survivors. I found some I wanted to attend and several that might benefit Gerry. However, he simply refused to go to any of the workshops I wasn't attending.

We spent the first morning orienting ourselves. I finally decided which sessions we should attend, ticking off the ones I felt were relevant to our situation.

Several hundred people attended this three-day conference. The numbers would be even greater if funding was available for everyone. Unfortunately, in most cases, the out-of-pocket expenses are absorbed solely by the survivor and the family. Sometimes registration can be subsidized through support groups, insurance, or Workers' Compensation. However, travel expenses, which can be quite costly, are not usually covered.

Many of the people attending the conference had sustained a brain injury and some had physical impairments as well. Gerry could not get beyond that. It upset him to see people with physical challenges, and he was disgusted when anyone was disruptive in the workshops.

The featured speakers included clinical professors, doctors, neuropsychologist, therapists, practitioners, researchers and sometimes family members.

I recall one particular workshop we attended on the last day of the conference that was directed by Al Condeluci, a strikingly handsome doctor from Pennsylvania. He was a phenomenal speaker and I enjoyed the lecture immensely. Also in attendance was a man in his twenties. The young man continually interrupted this speaker, offering the audience details of his own injuries whether they pertained to the doctor's presentation or not. The doctor was not at all fazed by the young man's interruptions. Instead, he gently but briefly acknowledged the young man's comments and moved on. Gerry was frustrated by this activity. At first, he sighed and shuffled in his seat. Eventually, he began tugging at my sleeve.

"God! What a jerk!" he said, in a loud whisper.

"S-s-h, Gerry. He'll hear you," I whispered back.

"I don't care. He's a jerk."

Other people in the room began to shift in their seats, casting glances our way. I was embarrassed. Then I felt guilty for being embarrassed. The young man was behaving no differently than anyone else, except that he didn't have any control over his reactions.

"Do you want to leave?"

"Yeah. I've had enough of this shit," Gerry replied, getting up and heading for the exit. He didn't notice that the noise he made leaving the room was interrupting Dr. Condeluci in the same way that young man was.

Warmth tingled beneath my cheeks. I nodded apologetically to the speaker before leaving the room. By the time I got into the hallway, Gerry was sitting on a plush love seat with his head cupped in his hands.

"Are you okay?" I asked, sitting down beside him. Suddenly I regretted bringing him to the conference. He wasn't ready.

A Change of Mind

"Why? Why are you doing this to me?" he asked with tears in his eyes. "I'm not like these people. They're disgusting!"

"I'm sorry, Honey. This wasn't done to hurt you. I thought we could learn something. Maybe we are not ready."

"I'll never be ready," he bellowed. A woman exiting from the nearby restroom stared in our direction. Gerry was quick to react. "Why do people stare at me? Can't they just leave me alone?" He did not comprehend that people would naturally be taken aback by the sight of a grown man emotionally distraught in a hotel lobby.

Under the circumstances, I saw no point in our staying at the conference any longer. Gerry agreed. Both of us were exhausted. Everywhere we looked, we saw displays about seatbelts, bicycle helmets, private rehabilitation, companies and support services. This, combined with the ongoing workshops, made it a tremendous amount of information to take in at one time.

After arriving back at my sister's, we visited for a while with John and Debby but took the luxury of turning in early that night. Gerry quickly fell asleep. I laid there, tossing and turning. I went over and over in my mind how Gerry had been so upset over the people he saw during the day. I couldn't help but wonder if and when he would get through a full day without crying.

Sometime in the middle of the night, Gerry awoke from a terrible nightmare. I felt as though I had just fallen asleep when his moaning startled me. My eyes pierced the darkness trying to focus on his face. His hands were clasping his head.

"What's wrong, Gerry?" My hand grazed his moisture drenched chest. "Are you okay?"

"My Dad - my Dad was here to get me. He wanted me to go home with him."

My heart skipped a beat. Gerry's father had been dead for nearly 17 years.

"Honey, it was just a dream. Your Dad is dead. Don't you remember?"

"I know he is dead. But he was here. I swear - he was right here."

"Do you want me to turn on the light?"

"No, no. Just hold me. I'm so scared," he sobbed.

I slipped my arm beneath him, cradling his head on my shoulders. It wasn't long before he settled down and fell back to sleep. However, I was wide-awake, recalling his words over and over. He didn't believe it was a dream. And neither did I.

Three weeks earlier I too had had a disturbing dream. I was walking down the street. Coming toward me was my brother Brian. I knew he was dead and so did he. Nonetheless, I approached him, smiling and soaking in the vision of him dressed in an outfit he often wore - blue jeans, a blue plaid shirt, and brown Hush Puppy shoes. He was smoking a cigarette. His hair and mustache were a rich black and his skin a perfect olive tone.

When I was within touching distance, he said, "Hi, Janelle. How are you doing?" Then he walked past me. I turned. "Brian - wait! Aren't you going to tell me what is going to happen to us now?"

Calmly, Brian replied. "Now, Janelle, you know if you want to know that, then you have to come and sit up here with God and all the other angels. But what I can tell you is that you are going to be just fine."

He faded away. And I woke up.

There was no doubt this was more than a dream about Brian. It was a terrible premonition about Gerry. Naturally, I didn't breathe a word of it to Gerry. My Mother was the only person I told about the dream. Now, with Gerry's dream, I was even more certain there was danger ahead.

During our flight home, I analyzed the two dreams in my head. They haunted me. Something was wrong, but I just couldn't put my finger on it. Gerry was different. He was withdrawn and sickly looking. Even after we arrived home, he wasn't his usual carefree self. After putting the girls to bed, I encouraged Gerry to go to bed too. I didn't know what else to do but entice him into getting some rest. Gerry flipped through the TV channels on the television in our bedroom while

I made notes about the brain injury conference and his dream in my journal.

Gerry started chatting about the girls, turning over on his side to face me. As he did, his face paled. He gasped. "Oh, my God! I've got a cramp in my chest!"

A warning flag shot up in my head. Book and pen dropped onto my lap. "Should I call the doctor?"

"No, no. It's okay." Gerry pressed on his chest with one hand and used the other to seize my wrist.

"Gerry, I think we should call Dr. Quandt," I persisted.

He wouldn't have anything to do with it. It was just a cramp. Notifying the doctor would be a waste of time. I had a different opinion. The dreams continued to haunt me. Periodically over the past five months, Gerry had complained of feeling short of breath. When I took him to see Dr. Quandt about it, he denied ever having difficulty breathing. My fears soon took the shape of certainty. Something was wrong with his heart. I just knew it.

Soon after the cramping, he was sound asleep. Not me. I lay beside him, watching and studying every detail. His eyes, eyelashes, brows, nose, hair, cheeks and mouth. I told myself if Gerry wasn't going to see the doctor then I should. The overwhelming fear that something was going to happen to him was beginning to cripple me. I had to get a grip on myself.

Monday and Tuesday were consumed with my watching Gerry's every move. No matter how hard I tried, I could not stop asking him if he was feeling okay. It annoyed him. But the terrifying look on his face when he had the chest pain was etched into my mind.

Wednesday, October 24, 1990. Gerry looked terrible. His skin was gray and taut. He didn't want to talk. He didn't even want to eat. Nothing sparked an interest in him - not even the fact that he had the day off from being with his caregiver.

Our friend, Judie Johnson, planned to spend the day with him while I went into town to work. It was near the month's end and I had a stack of paperwork to catch up on. Judie and I thought Gerry might enjoy going for lunch with her and then into town to do some shopping. Gerry kept saying he was too tired. He wanted me to call Judie and cancel for him. Finally, I asked him if he would go with Judie because I had heard an advertisement on the radio for a lady style mountain bike. I suggested he could buy it and we would put it away for Christmas to give to Myriah if he thought the bike was worth the price. This excited him, so he agreed to go.

It was difficult for me to leave him that morning. He seemed so fragile and vulnerable. It felt almost like leaving a small child with a baby sitter. I knew I had to get my work done, but still the guilt washed over me.

It wasn't as though we were completely separated. Gerry phoned me three times within the first hour while I was at a client's office. After he saw the bike, he had Judie bring him to the office so he could tell me about it. An hour later, he phoned to say he had paid for the bike and Judie would have Lloyd pick it up on Friday. This time he started to cry.

There was no reason for the tears. He missed me and said he couldn't wait to see me again. It was a tough plea to turn aside. What was the use? I couldn't concentrate anyway.

"How about I meet you and Judie for lunch at the pub?" I suggested. "After lunch we can go home and then we'll walk down to the school at three o'clock to meet the girls."

He could not believe what he was hearing. "But what about all your work?"

"Trust me. It will be here tomorrow. If you need me at home, I'll come."

"Yes - yes, I do," he sobbed into the telephone.

When I arrived at the neighborhood pub some thirty minutes later, I spotted Judie at a table near the window. From where she was sitting I could see the roof of our house.

"Hi. Gerry's in the restroom," explained Judie, lighting a cigarette. "Is he okay, Janelle? He looks awfully gray and he is so tired today."

A Change of Mind

Keeping a watchful eye for his return, I quickly filled Judie in about the chest pains he had on Sunday night and how tired Gerry had been feeling since.

"Maybe you better call Dr. Quandt."

"I tried. Gerry won't let me. Besides, Dr. Quandt probably can't do anything on the basis of one chest pain. At most he could only monitor him. However, Gerry has a scheduled appointment on Friday. I'm going to ask to speak privately with him. It really has me scared."

We were already ordering our food when Gerry came back to the table. He did look tired. The chair scraped across the wood planks as he sat down, pulling it in. I smiled and patted his shoulder. He didn't say a word. By the time our food arrived he wanted to go home to bed. Judie and I convinced him to eat a little bit. And a little was all he ate.

I could tell from his expression that he was more depressed than he had been in the morning. Normally, my taking the afternoon off work would have delighted him. Today, it didn't seem to matter.

After lunch, we made the short drive home and then went for a walk. Our conversation circled around the kids, renovations to our house and Christmas. General stuff. There was nothing said that should have upset him. But it did. He started crying. He cried and cried. Even going to the school to get the girls didn't help. By the time we got home, his crying was uncontrollable. By four o'clock, I was beside myself. I decided to give him some Ativan to help relax him. Then I suggested he lie down for a nap. He agreed, but only if our youngest daughter Dale sat with him. I felt sorry for her. She was only ten and instead of watching TV or going outside to play with friends, she was being asked to baby-sit her father while I prepared dinner. She did not seem to mind, though.

What a roller coaster the afternoon had been! I hated this new life. Why couldn't I make it better? Not just for me, but for Gerry too. The pieces to the puzzle were scattered everywhere. Nothing fit into place any more.

Gerry's nap seemed to do the trick. He came downstairs to dinner looking and sounding like a new man. Happy, talkative and incredibly hungry. It was amazing - and confusing. The events of the day were like a storm passing through our valley.

My shoulders felt heavy as I set the dinner table. Gerry was happy, but I felt irritable. I was exhausted. Pressure was building up inside of me. I didn't know how much more I could take before I would start falling apart.

As I was doing the dishes after supper, I received a telephone call from a friend in the village. Naturally, the topic was Gerry but this man was concerned for all of us. The warmth in his voice and his offer to help in any way put me over the edge. I choked. Then I collapsed into tears, like a paper bag breaking from carrying a heavy load. I was so upset I had to hang up. Unbeknownst to me, Gerry had been standing behind me the entire time. My hand covered my mouth. Oh God! I didn't want him to see me like this.

"You're crying," he said, with the biggest smile I'd ever seen. I was immobilized. Gerry stepped forward and wrapped his arms around me, pulling my head onto his chest. "I haven't seen you cry since the accident. I didn't think you felt sad for what I've lost."

"Of course I feel sad, Gerry," I said, looking up into his eyes. "But what good would it do if I broke down all the time, too?" Feeling defensive, I tried to push him away.

"Come here. Let me hold you. I want to be your husband again. I want to look after you," he said, pulling me close again. It felt so good to be in his arms. I felt like his wife again, instead of his nurse. His soothing words made me realize that my keeping a stiff upper lip all the time had diminished his self-respect. He had missed being my nurturing and protective husband. Gerry wiped my eyes, promptly reminding me I had a meeting in thirty minutes with the Ladies Auxiliary at the village fire hall.

The last thing I wanted to do was attend a strategy session on fundraising. In the first place, I didn't have the strength. Secondly, I had not made arrangements for anyone to come and sit with Gerry and the girls.

"Come on. I want to look after the girls myself. I want to be a father to them again. Please!" he pleaded, convincingly. I wanted to let him try.

"Well, I'm coming home at nine o'clock. No matter what! Even if the meeting isn't finished – I'm coming home. That way you won't be alone after the kids go to bed. Are you sure you will be okay?"

"Yes, I'm sure. Besides the fire hall is at the end of the street. You will be two minutes away if I need you."

"Okay. But remember, I'm coming home at nine. Agreed?"

"Agreed!" He hugged me hard. Twenty minutes later we stood at the door kissing goodbye. My eyes filled with tears. Something felt ominous, but I also felt I had to go and let him try.

My mind wandered all through the meeting. It was a relief when it came to a close around 8:45 p.m. I had no intention of staying, but Marg Kean poured coffee for everyone, including me.

"Janelle, can you stay for a cup?" she asked.

Looking at my watch, I replied, "Sure. I've got 15 minutes before I'm due home." Dropping my notebook to the floor, I stood up, approaching the counter. Surely he would have called if something went wrong. My feet suddenly stopped moving. Everything in my mind went blank. My ears closed off the world. All I could hear was a strange voice inside my head shouting, "Phone home! Phone home! Phone home!"

The words thumped inside my skull. A flutter of heartbeats pounded in my chest. No one seemed to notice me rushing to the phone. My fingers couldn't dial the numbers to our house fast enough. Finally, I succeeded. It began to ring. It rang and rang. Something was wrong. I could feel it, but I was too terrified to hang up. At last, someone answered! I could barely make out Gerry's voice. He sounded terribly distressed.

"Gerry … it's me … Janelle! What's wrong?!"

"I'm having those pains in my chest again. Oh, God! I'm going to die!" He was shouting into the telephone.

"I'm on my way," I shouted back into the mouthpiece. The receiver dropped into the cradle. All eyes were on me when I turned around.

"Marg, call an ambulance! Gerry's having a heart attack!" I ordered. My legs raced to the door and down the stairwell. Our house was only two minutes away yet something told me those might be minutes I didn't have.

The station wagon had barely stopped before I shut off the ignition. My mouth was bone dry. Where were the kids? The door flew open into our kitchen. It was empty. There was no sign of Gerry or the girls. I called out their names over the hum of the dishwasher. No one - no answer.

"Gerry?" I called again. I realized that he must be up in the bedroom. My legs climbed the stairs two at a time. I braced myself against the door of the master bedroom.

"Oh, God!" I screamed. Gerry was lying sideways across our bed with his jeans down around his ankles. He had his housecoat on part way.

"Help me! I'm dying!" he screamed, obviously in horrific pain.

"Honey, don't say that. You won't die. The ambulance is on the way." I placed my open hand on his chest and then his face. Beads of perspiration trickled down his face and neck.

He was definitely having a heart attack.

"What's happening to me?" he screamed.

"Gerry, try to stay calm. You need to be calm. The ambulance is on the way." I looked around for the kids. "Gerry, where are the kids?" He did not respond. "Where are the girls, Gerry?"

"Oh, God, the pain."

"I know, Honey. I know." I stroked his drenched hair. "Honey, can you tell me where the kids are?"

"Ah, downstairs," I knew downstairs meant in the basement. That's where the television was. I wondered why they hadn't heard him screaming.

It had only been in recent weeks that emergency calls had to be dispatched through a 911 Call Centre. Prior to that, emergency calls were directed to our local volunteer firemen and first aid attendants who would have been called and on the scene within minutes. I had no idea how long it would take for the ambulance to come from the city to our house in the village. The hospital was at least eighteen to twenty minutes away by car.

The phone rang and startled me. I hurled myself across the bed to get it before the kids picked up the extension in the basement.

"Hello?"

"Is this the Breese residence?" asked a strange male voice.

"Yes," I replied, somewhat impatient.

"Mrs. Breese? This is the ambulance service. Someone requested an ambulance to attend your home. What seems to be the problem?"

"What? You mean they haven't been dispatched yet? It's my husband - he's having a heart attack! Please, we need help!"

"They are on the way, Mrs. Breese. But I need some information to pass on to them."

His questions seemed to take an eternity to answer. It was difficult to concentrate on what he was saying because Gerry was screaming in the background. At the same time I was trying to keep an eye on the bedroom door in case the girls came upstairs.

As soon as I hung up the telephone, I dialed Judie and Lloyd. They lived only minutes away. Then I called my mother.

"Mom … Mom …" I burst into tears. "Mom, meet me at the hospital. It's Gerry. I think he's having a heart attack." My body shook.

The next thing I remember was dialing Nathan's number. Three times I tried to call him. Each time, the same young male voice answered. I thought he kept saying that I had reached the Coast Lakeside, a local hotel. It didn't make any sense. "How could I dial the same wrong number, three times in a row?" I screamed out loud, slamming the phone down.

Gerry was suddenly trying to get up from the bed. He made a funny noise and fell backwards. Urine sprayed over him and the bed. Fluids came up through his nose. He clenched his teeth. The blue eyes I loved were fixed straight ahead. His body went stiff.

My shrill voice broke the silence in the room. I stamped my feet and then collapsed beside the bed. "Oh, my God. Where is the ambulance!?"

On one hand, time seemed to be moving at a snail's pace. Yet at the same time, Gerry's life was passing quickly. I wanted to vomit. Someone had to help us. I staggered to the stairs and ran down to the kitchen and out the front door. No one heard my cry for help. None of the women from the meeting had followed me.

An incredulous thought popped into my head. "That guy wasn't saying that I had reached the Coast Lakeside. He was saying Nathan's AT the Coast Lakeside!"

I dashed to the kitchen phone and forced my trembling fingers to dial the RCMP detachment. "Who is this? Who is this?" I shouted into the phone as soon as I heard the man's voice say, "Good evening …"

"Constable A. J. McKinnon."

"God! A.J. It's Gerry. He's had a heart attack. I don't know CPR and he's not breathing. Please help us!"

"Janelle? Janelle, did you call an ambulance?"

"They're on their way. But I need someone to get my brother, Nathan. He's at the Coast Lakeside."

"Okay, I'm on my way!" The telephone line went dead.

"Mommy … Mommy, what's wrong? Where's Daddy?" Both Myriah and Dale were standing behind me. They had heard me screaming into the telephone.

My arms reached out for them. "Oh, girls, I'm so sorry. I think Daddy has had a heart attack." Their little faces twisted with panic.

"Where is he?" screeched Myriah, her eyes darting around the room.

"Upstairs. You can't go up there. Come outside with me." I tried to guide them to the door.

"No! No! Call 911! Mommy, call 911! You have to do something," shouted Dale, pulling her little hand from mine.

"I did, Dale. I did. They're coming." I explained, herding the two outside clothed in pajamas.

From the front steps I could see the fire truck's lights flashing spots of red against the night sky. Marg must have called the volunteer firemen as well. We huddled on the porch waiting for the truck to stop. Men clad in yellow coats and black boots jumped from the truck. The first fireman I recognized was Chuck Simonin.

"He's not breathing, Chuck! He's not breathing!" I yelled, charging toward him.

Chuck held a hand firmly on my shoulder and asked me where Gerry was. The firemen followed my directions, storming into the house carrying a medical kit.

My whole body trembled until my legs finally gave out sending me tumbling to the ground. I felt incredibly cold and began to shiver. My teeth chattered so hard that I couldn't speak. The saliva in my mouth dried up leaving me parched. I was going into shock.

Cars slowed down as they passed our house, knowing the fire trucks meant something was really wrong. Marg Kean arrived, coming to sit with me on the grass. Chuck wrapped a gray army blanket around my shoulders.

"My k-k-kids. W-w-w-here are the girls?" I chattered, suddenly aware they were nowhere to be seen.

Chuck replied, "They're okay. Judie Johnson took them inside."

I scrambled to my feet insisting, "I-I n-need to go to them."

The girls were huddled together in the darkened living room. I joined them. From the sofa we could see directly through the kitchen and up the stairs leading to the master bedroom. In silence, we sat, our arms linked – waiting.

The front door suddenly burst open. Nathan and Cy Kelly rushed in. I stood up to explain. The words wouldn't come. Cy wrapped his arms around my shoulders. I didn't realize he was preventing me from seeing up the stairs. The sounds of footsteps and voices coming down caught my attention. I tried to turn around, but Cy held me firmly. Nathan took my hand, saying, "You don't need to see this." My eyes were closed. I concentrated on the voices. A man's voice methodically gave instructions.

"One … two … three…"

The numbers pierced my heart. Reality took hold. I pulled hard trying to free myself from Cy's grip. Both Cy and Nathan held my arms tight. Overwhelmed with grief, I fell to the floor, sobbing.

"Come on, Janelle. We have to get to the hospital," Nathan said. They helped me up. Judie offered to take the girls home with her. "They should come to the hospital with me," I said. Judie disagreed, and I didn't have time to argue. They were crying when I kissed them goodbye. Charlie Bomford, the local volunteer fire chief opened Nathan's car door for me.

"Please find Danny, Charlie. Tell him his brother needs him." Living in a small town has its advantages. Everyone knows everyone and where he or she lives.

"We'll see he gets to the hospital," Charlie replied.

The attendants loaded Gerry into the back of the ambulance. Someone slammed the doors closed. Red lights flashed as the vehicle sped out of the driveway.

Nathan and I pulled out behind the emergency vehicle which was soon out of sight. The thirteen mile trip to the hospital seemed endless.

Tears soaked my shirt. There had been no time to say goodbye.

A Tribute

By the time Nathan and I arrived at the hospital, the parking lot was dotted with blue and white police cars. The ambulance was parked in front of the emergency entrance, its doors still open. Mom and Rebecca were waiting for us on the sidewalk. They quickly followed me as I hurried past them into the hospital waiting area. The nurse on duty was the same one who had been there the night of Gerry's accident. She recognized me immediately and moved quickly from behind the counter to greet me.

"Mrs. Breese, why don't you have a seat in the family room? There are a lot of people working on your husband right now, so it will be a while before we know anything."

The waiting room was the same family room we had waited in when Gerry was injured. Within minutes, the room was filled with the same family, friends and police officers who had been with us on that fateful night five months prior.

Each person I spoke with offered words of encouragement. It was only me who insisted that death had come. I had been right there with Gerry. I knew it was over. Instinct told me there was no way he could have possibly survived.

The wait seemed endless. When Dr. Quandt and Nathan finally approached us, the sorrowful look in their eyes confirmed the certainty that Gerry's fight was over. Dr. Quandt had barely finished saying he was sorry when I charged, "He's dead, isn't he?!"

He rested a hand on my shoulder. "Yes. Yes, he is."

The reality of our loss spread like wildfire through the room. Some raced outside for fresh air while others clung to one another as though the nightmare would end if they hung on long enough. But it didn't.

It broke my heart when Rebecca and Judie brought Myriah and Dale to the hospital. They looked like Siamese twins when they walked into the room, their little bodies pressed against one another.

The few people in the room with us left as soon as the girls walked in. The last person to leave was Hughie Winters who slowly closed the door behind him.

Dale's little hands grasped her big sister's arm. Myriah had her eyes fixed on mine, chewing one of her thumbnails. My arms reached out for them. Myriah fired her worst fear at me, just as I had minutes before at Dr. Quandt.

"He's dead, isn't he? Daddy's dead!"

No words came to mind that could possibly ease their shock. I could only nod my head. Their two little heads bowed. Sorrowful cries filled the room. I held their trembling bodies close to mine.

* * *

On October 30, 1990, at 10:00 a.m., over 250 Royal Canadian Mounted Police Officers from across Alberta and British Columbia lined up in front of Penticton's prestigious Trade and Convention Center, the only sizeable building to hold the anticipated large crowd. News reporters from the local paper and television station waited in the parking lot.

Nearly eight hundred individuals flowed through the doors. They were family, friends, Gerry's work mates, business associates and perfect strangers. All of them had come to pay their respects.

The black limousine that my daughters and I rode in slowed to a stop at the curb. The tinted windows prevented spectators from seeing us. However, we had a clear view of the groups huddled together bracing themselves from the bitterly cold wind that ripped through coats and sent the dried autumn leaves scurrying down the sidewalk.

A familiar face approached the car – Constable Jan Egger – a co-worker who Gerry unreservedly respected. Her husband Don and their two daughters, Shannon and Becky, had become close family friends.

"Hi, Janelle," Jan said, opening the car door. "I'm your personal escort today. If you or the girls need anything, I'll take care of it." Our hands linked as she helped me from the car.

Just then Nathan approached, dressed in his sheriff's uniform. He

A Change of Mind

rested his hand on Jan's red serge coat and asked, "Are you okay, Janelle? The reporters are here."

"I see that, Nathan. I don't mind really, but please ask them to refrain from taking pictures inside. They can take as many as they want before and after the service, just not during."

"No problem," he said, confidently, as he spun on his heels to take charge and deliver my message.

I finally gave way to the tears. My arms were wrapped protectively around my daughters as they walked on either side of me. How terribly frightening this must be for them, I thought.

This wasn't just saying goodbye to my beloved husband. It was saying goodbye to our life as a family. A huge void had been created. There was absolutely nothing I could do.

Our family and close friends gathered in a private waiting area. We were to be the last people seated before the police officers escorted Gerry's flag-draped casket to the front. As I waited for the signal to start, I reflected on the preparation for Gerry's funeral.

First, the funeral home had employed Jeff Nielson, the man who had worked alongside Jake Wiens to resuscitate Gerry on the night of his accident. Second, the Chaplain scheduled to conduct the service was Tim Schroeder, the same "Tim" who mysteriously appeared at the Kelowna Hospital the night Gerry was injured. The third coincidence was Ann Mortifee. Ann, a very talented singer, was Chuck Simonin's sister-in-law. In early September, Gerry had had his caregiver take him to visit Chuck. Ann happened to be visiting Chuck and his wife Mary at the same time. Ann and Gerry had a wonderful conversation about life and spirituality. Her words moved Gerry to a far greater understanding of God and the power of His love. When Gerry died, Chuck contacted Ann. She graciously offered to perform as soloist for his service.

There was little doubt these people had been placed in our lives for very definite reasons. The only regret was Gerry had never had the opportunity to meet Tim or Jeff or to personally thank them. He wanted to, but at the time, he and I felt he wasn't strong enough to handle an emotional reunion. Therefore, having Jeff and Tim participate in Gerry's funeral seemed to bring about a sense of completion for me.

Nathan offered a tearful eulogy. His words soothed the deep wounds that not only the girls and I felt but for those also felt by my family and our many friends. Ann's angelic voice sent "Amazing Grace" floating across the room to provide everyone the opportunity to let their deep sadness spill forth.

A procession of police motorcycles led the cars from the convention center to the cemetery. Civilians and officers lined the walkway offering silent respect as we passed by. The hearse took Gerry on his final tour of the city.

The limos stopped closest to the graveside. We pulled on coats against the brisk cold wind sweeping from the nearby lake. Vehicles slowly turned into the cemetery. Headlights from other cars, that were unable to get into the grounds because there was no more room, could be seen for a mile down the road.

Gerry was being buried two spaces over from Ruth. The crowd gathered around. Many had stood here only two weeks earlier to say goodbye to Ruth. Her floral arrangements still graced the ground.

Slowly, Myriah, Dale and I walked across the grass. Flowers laid at the edge of the astroturf hid the mound of dirt that would cover Gerry.

The pallbearers carefully rested the royal blue casket on the straps that would lower Gerry to his final resting place. The spray of white pink-tipped roses swayed in the cold wind. Three pink roses in the center represented Myriah, Dale and me. I couldn't help smiling. Those three flowers seemed lower than the rest, sheltered and protected from the bitter elements. A sign that we too would have the protection we needed.

For as far as I could see, red coats and brown Stetsons dotted the leaf-covered grass. Many of the officers were men that I had not seen in years. Others I had never met, but they came to pay their respects to a fallen officer. A silence hovered as we waited for the Chaplain to begin.

Tim offered words of encouragement and peace to replenish us. Heads turned down. Sniffles swept through the crowd. I was so proud. This was a celebration of Gerry's life. More than anyone else I knew, Gerry deserved recognition for what he gave unconditionally to his family and to this community.

One by one, the officers filed in front of Gerry's casket to face my daughters and me. With all the control they could muster, one by one, they clicked their heels and regally lifted a gloved hand to their Stetson to give one final salute. Truly a tribute fit for an officer of the law.

A Change of Mind

The Journey Ahead

The three months following Gerry and Ruth's funerals were a downward spiral. Each new day meant facing our routine without him at our side. Many everyday tasks that I had previously taken for granted were now excruciatingly painful - like doing the grocery shopping alone or cooking meals without him at my side to handle the barbecue. Most painful of all was setting the table for three instead of four.

My family, as did Gerry's family and our close friends, kept a watchful eye on the three of us. Some days that was enough to pull us through. Other days, no matter what anyone did, I cried so hard that it felt like I could turn myself inside out.

Life without Gerry was so incredibly lonely. After all, he wasn't someone that I had spent only a few years with. We had been a couple for 17 years – half of my 34 years had been with him.

Myriah and Dale missed him too. He wasn't there to watch TV with them. He wasn't there to make his incredible butter drenched popcorn. No more bear hugs. No more kisses on the forehead. No more sitting on Daddy's knee.

My first major decision was to move to a house in town where we would be closer to family. I just couldn't take coming home to that house. I knew I would be tortured by the memories of what had taken place that night. But also, I expected to see him looking out the kitchen window or perched on the front steps with a cold beer in hand each time I pulled into the driveway.

Our new home was located in a newer subdivision. Even though we had all of Gerry's pictures and RCMP paraphernalia, we didn't have to fight the expectation that he should be right around the corner. With each passing day, the activity of visitors lessened. Many of our friends stopped calling and invitations stopped coming. We had to face the reality of life by ourselves. He just wasn't coming back.

I missed him. I missed my brother Brian. I missed Ruth.

Three of the most important people in my life were gone – all during the past year – all due to brain injuries. The fragility of life rocked me to the very core. I battled a deep sense of mortality. The feeling of abandonment was so intense and painful that I longed to be with them – especially with Gerry.

It was nearing Christmas before I really began to face my feelings. Naturally, holiday celebrations were nothing I wanted to be a part of. Shopping was unpleasant. Putting up the Christmas tree seemed formidable. However, a simple song changed that.

While waiting for the girls to come home from school one afternnon, I sat in the living room listening to the radio. Like so many times before, tears streamed down my cheeks as I thought about Christmas morning without him. I wanted to run – get on a plane with the girls and fly to a country that did not celebrate Christmas. Somewhere – as long as it was anywhere but here.

A message came to me over the radio. It was a song performed by a male artist. I had not heard his name or most of the song. All I tuned into was this:

... Daddy's gone, but Christmas must go on, because the little ones need the memories.

I sobbed. How selfish of me! Of course the girls needed to know it was okay to go on. We had to celebrate Christmas, just as we had in the past. We just had to find ways to make it extra special.

On Christmas Eve, the girls and I went to the cemetery to place flowers on Gerry's grave. A thin blanket of crisp snow covered the ground. We had put it off as long as possible. Now the sky had given way to dusk. Tiny decorated Christmas trees were scattered throughout the property. These tokens of love marked the visits of other families who had come to fill the void left by a loved one passing on.

It was one of the hardest days in my life. The three of us stood in silence. We couldn't avoid looking at each other. The moment our eyes connected, the tears began to flow. I reached into my pocket retrieving Kleenex for all of us. If nothing else, I had learned to be prepared.

"While we are here today, girls, I wanted to talk to you about your Dad and me," I said, trying to keep my voice steady. Both girls stood silent. Myriah bit down on her bottom lip, folding her arms over her heavy jacket. Dale dabbed her eye with Kleenex.

"I want you both to understand how much Dad and I loved each other and loved both of you. We didn't take our marriage lightly. It meant a great deal to both of us." Slowly and steadily I described the expectations we had for marriage to the girls and how they had truly been a blessing in the communion of our life together.

Once again, I reached into my pocket. This time, instead of Kleenex, I drew out two velvet ring cases. The girls had not noticed that I had removed my wedding rings earlier in the day. My fingers trembled as I pushed open the lids. My diamond engagement ring and wedding band were in one, Gerry's wedding band in the other.

Tenderly, I handed Myriah my set and Dale her Dad's.

"What makes this day so difficult for me," I said, "is not that it's Christmas or that Daddy won't be here. It's that I realize I am not married to him anymore."

My voice shattered. Silence fell once again between us.

Dale moved closer to me, snuggling into my arms. Her sobs cut deep. I reached for Myriah, pulling her into our hug.

"I miss him," she wept.

"I know you do, Honey," I soothed. "He knows too. But you have to know that whatever you do, Daddy's watching over you and he'll be there to protect us. That's why I want you to have our wedding rings. They are a symbol of where you came from and a reminder of the love we had as a family."

Our embrace tightened. Alone, we stood grieving, supporting one another. My eyes closed. Just as I knew he would be, there he was – his memory flourishing, offering us strength.

"Are you okay, Mom?" asked Dale, her black mittens smoothing away the tears on her cheeks.

"Oh, God, I just miss him. I'm not ready to be without him," I sobbed. A warmth flowed through me, as his memory surfaced in my mind. Holding tightly together, we slowly moved to the car and drove home.

I tucked the girls into bed later that night. Once they were asleep, I placed their filled Christmas stockings on the bottom of their beds, just as Gerry and I had always done on Christmas Eve. I stayed up as long as I could, as had become my routine, so when I went to bed I wouldn't have to fight for sleep.

The bed was so big and cold when I got in. All that had been no longer was. I closed my eyes allowing the tears to trickle down my face. I had wanted to be with him so much that, up to then, even death seemed inviting - particularly if that was the only way we could be together. But that night it was different.

After the trip to the cemetery, I didn't feel that way anymore. What I felt was a deep sense of responsibility for my children. For the first time in two months I knew, without a doubt, that I wanted to live and take care of them. I draped an arm over my head, pulling the covers tight. An overwhelming sense of guilt flooded my mind - guilt that I was choosing to survive and care for our daughters. Realizing how guilty I felt made me cry even harder.

Gerry's memory clearly formed in my mind. I could see him. I could feel him – his hair, his skin, his warm breath. "Oh God, Gerry! I'm sorry. I want to be with you, but I have to stay here with the girls," I said out loud, not caring if anyone heard. "I miss you, but they need me."

The sobs deepened. My chest heaved as the floodgates of grief released. Then, like magic, a sense of peace suddenly surrounded and comforted me. I stopped crying.

It was as though the memory of Gerry was holding me. He kissed me. I heard the soft whisper of his voice say, "It's okay, Honey, because I can't take you with me."

Epilogue

Many challenges were ahead of us the year following Gerry's death, the foremost being financial. During his recovery, Gerry's wages from the RCMP were uninterrupted, as though he was back working on the job. However, when he died, the autopsy concluded that the cause of his death was a heart attack due to heart disease. I was appalled to learn the autopsy results through the local newspaper. This conclusion, combined with the fact that his death occurred nearly six months after the accident, resulted in the RCMP rendering the shocking decision that Gerry's death was not duty related. This made a major difference in the amount of monthly pension that my daughters and I would receive.

When an officer's death is not duty related, the widow is entitled to a basic survivor's benefit. In my case, this was less than $600 per month for me and orphans' benefits of less than $155 per month for each of our daughters. If the officer's death is duty related, the survivors are entitled to an enhanced benefit - the equivalent of the officer's monthly net pay – for life.

I was shocked. It never occurred to me that his employer would find his death not related to the accident. Gerry's life insurance provided us with a mortgage free home and investments. However, it wasn't enough to sustain us with a decent monthly income, especially at my young age. Not only was my husband and the father of my children gone, but I now faced living on a drastically reduced income. The time spent with my daughters would suffer so I could work.

The personal injury claim initiated at the time of the accident was halted for similar reasons. The pathologist's report that Gerry's death was not related to the accident let the insurance company off the hook.

Something wasn't right. I could feel it. For nearly six months, I had watched Gerry live through pain and anguish. His confidence was shattered and his ability to make decisions was severely hampered. He would never have returned to work as a police officer and he sensed it. His parenting skills were greatly diminished as was his ability to participate in our marriage as an equal partner.

Granted, Gerry was considered a high risk for heart disease. He smoked, was slightly overweight, worked in a stressful job, and had a positive family history of heart disease. However, our family doctor was aware of these factors and had monitored Gerry's health accordingly. Gerry showed no indication of heart disease prior to the accident.

I began meeting with my lawyers, Gordon Marshall and Robin Adolphe, to determine a course of action. The plan of attack was a double action: one, to secure my income of an enhanced benefit from the RCMP; and, the other to sue the driver of the car on behalf of my daughters. The latter claim fell within the guidelines of the Family Compensation Act, which allows for the loss of love, care and guidance of a parent. Gordon and Robin warned me that the legal cost of overturning the pension decision and suing on behalf of my children could easily exceed the amount of life insurance money I had invested. We could lose. I didn't hesitate in making the decision. Not for one second. If I didn't pursue what I believed to be rightfully ours, I knew that I would live to regret it.

The family compensation claim was left in the capable hands of Robin Adolphe while I researched the effects of stress and heart disease. In doing so, I became fascinated with the findings of Dr. Dean Ornish from San Francisco, California. In his book, Reversing Heart Disease, Dr. Ornish refers to emotional stress, which he breaks into two basic categories: acute and chronic. To differentiate between acute and chronic stress, consider the following example: A child runs out in front of your moving car, you slam on the brakes and honk the horn. Your heart races and you breathe faster. Your grip tightens on the steering wheel. As frightening as this is, you eventually return to a relaxed state. Individuals under chronic stress never return to that baseline of relaxation. They can't, because they are hit with another stressful situation before recovering from the previous one.

In my opinion, Gerry was under chronic stress after his accident. He was never comfortable with the new person he was. Facing the possibility of not ever returning to work as a police officer was devastating to him and left him feeling inadequate and worthless.

Nothing I said or did, or that others did for that matter, seemed to ease these feelings for him. Gerry never returned to a baseline of relaxation after his accident. He couldn't. He no longer had that built in mechanism. My interpretation of Dr. Ornish's findings was that heart disease could be sped up when an individual was living under the condition of chronic stress. I also felt that in some cases this could be fatal.

Gerry's feelings of inferiority and worthlessness were prevalent the

A Change of Mind

morning of his death. I was confident that not only would a lay person accept this evidence in reading his journals, but a professional would too. If I could get someone to read them, that is.

For four months, I wrote and revised my research and conclusions on stress, heart disease and brain injuries into a six-page statement. Through this, I found that some of the warnings or indications of heart disease were also indicative of anxiety. Gerry always complained of being short of breath after the accident. The doctor and I believed he was experiencing anxiety or panic attacks. Extreme fatigue can be indicative of heart disease, but it is also very symptomatic of a brain injury. Survivors of brain injury can experience extreme fatigue, sometimes for very long periods of time or even years after sustaining a brain injury.

This statement went to my lawyers and the Bureau of Pension Advocates, an agency that, at no charge, worked to pursue my claim for full pension by challenging the Canadian Pension Commission.

My lawyers worked diligently to find a doctor to support my theory - not an easy task to say the least. It took two years and tremendous determination, but eventually they succeeded in finding a doctor in Boston, Massachusetts who openly supported me. His opinion was based in part on the journals kept by Gerry and myself. As far as he was concerned, there was no disputing the sadness, frustration and devastation recorded in Gerry's own handwriting.

On December 2, 1992, at a Pension Board Entitlement Hearing, my daughters and I were granted full pension from the RCMP. The children are to receive their benefits until the age of majority, or twenty-five, if attending school full-time. My pensions are for the rest of my life. The family compensation claim has been dealt with and received final approval through the courts. The amount of money each girl received is nominal; however, it contributed to their being able to purchase their first vehicle without having to borrow any money and to each purchase a computer.

The legal fees incurred originally exceeded $90,000. My lawyers graciously cut this in half, in recognition of my role in researching and documenting the effects of Gerry's injury and his cause of death.

A New Beginning

In late 1991, I met Lyle Biagioni. Lyle, a single father of three, is an angel in his own right. He encouraged me to go on living and to give myself permission to once again experience the joys of life, including falling in love. We married on December 26, 1992. The blending of our families brought the grand total of children to five: Myriah, Dale, Matthew, Bradley & Sarah.

Lyle's unconditional love and encouragement of my passion to companion families and individuals affected by brain injury was instrumental in the completion of my first book: <u>Head Injuries: The Silent Epidemic</u>. Until I met Lyle, I doubted the value of my story and lacked confidence to complete the manuscript, which had come to collect dust for nearly a year. I am eternally grateful to him and our children for their unwavering support and enthusiasm in concluding this project.

Following the release of my book, I was invited to participate on the Board of Directors for the South Okanagan Similkameen Brain Injury Society (SOSBIS). My connection with SOSBIS provided many opportunities to bond with families and individuals living with the outcome of acquired brain injury. They provided me with insight and affirmed the need to develop educational material that would assist them and others in rebuilding their lives. The membership of SOSBIS, in particular John, Ken, Keith, Brenda, Carol, Darrin, Harriet, Phil, and Mike have inspired me with their courage, dedication and commitment to build a stronger community for those living with the outcome of acquired brain injury.

In 2001, I relocated my family to accept a permanent staff position with the Brain Association of BC (BABC) in Victoria, British Columbia. During my employment with BABC, I had the privilege of meeting families, survivors and professionals across the country who strive to raise the public and government's awareness on the effects of living with acquired brain injury. Shortly after our move, I also undertook a commitment to complete a Certificate in Death and Grief Studies through the Center for Loss and Life Transition at Colorado State University in Fort Collins, Colorado. As my studies will conclude later this year, I have resigned from my position at BABC to pursue my long-standing dream of opening a Grief and Loss Retreat Center for bereaved families and families affected by catastrophic events. Please visit my website www.soulwriter.com for updates on these plans.

Hope Begins with a Heartbeat

I felt a profound sense of hope when I was told that although Gerry's injuries were life-threatening and he had gone into cardiac arrest at the scene, bystanders had successfully resuscitated him and his heart was beating strong. It was some time before I asked or even thought about what the long term effects of his injuries might be. Just knowing he was alive meant everything to me. It meant our family was still four – not three. It meant I was married – not single. It meant he survived – and I thought it meant we as a family would too.

Although the news was bad – he had extensive bruising, multiple broken bones and a severe closed head injury – I quickly and eagerly assumed the role of caregiver, operating with the mindset that as long as I was there for him, that as long as I was the one to take care of him – he would be just fine.

There were a myriad of details to take care of in the immediate hours following the crash. He was being moved to another hospital some sixty minutes away by car. His life was in a fragile state so I needed to travel with him and planned to stay with him until his condition could be upgraded from critical and he could be transferred to our home community hospital. This meant that I would be gone from home for an indefinite period of time. I had to make quick decisions – would I take the girls with me or not? If not, where would they stay? How would they get to school – or should they even go? What about my bookkeeping clients who were dependent on my payroll services and had staff to pay in the next seven days? These details and others, right down to who would care for the family dog, water the grass, and generally keep an eye on our house were overwhelming. However, I did what I had to do and made the decisions decisively and quickly.

Over the next few weeks I had more decisions to make about his care, rehabilitation, and the future legal proceedings. There were communications with senior officers of the RCMP on what he would need for care once I brought him home and even preliminary discussions on whether it would be possible for him to return to work as a police officer.

I juggled tasks, meetings, telephone calls and correspondence and successfully managed to organize and orchestrate his care, the needs and schedule of our children, the needs of my clients and the proceedings for a legal case with skill and precision.

The days moved into weeks and those weeks snowballed into months. All the while, I ran a tight ship and kept "it" all together for his sake, the sake of our children and I suppose, for the sake of everyone around us.

I handled the bank accounts, paid the household bills, managed my home-based business, parented the girls, communicated with family and friends and advocated for his medical and legal rights.

I slept when he slept – about 3 hours a night in total. When he napped during the day, I used the time to do laundry, prepare the next meal, write a letter, make notes on his condition, clean the house, help the girls with their homework, and respond to the endless pile of telephone messages inquiring about his condition.

In the five and one-half months Gerry lived following the crash, I readily gave up on having a solid night's sleep, enjoying a leisurely dinner, having lunch with a friend, or indulging in a quiet soak in the tub and even my usual Sunday morning down time when I stayed in my housecoat and drank a full pot of coffee while reading a stack of magazines or a good book. In essence – I gave up me.

My personal needs became secondary to everything else. All that seemed to matter was getting him through the day and finding some way to hold everything together. I quickly fell into the trap that no one – not anyone – could care for him or make any of the decisions the way I could. I didn't want a nurse to help with his care. I didn't want anyone to fill my role as mom. And I didn't want to disappoint my clients by not providing the same standard of service they had become accustomed to receiving from me.

I didn't feel anything. I had no self-awareness. I didn't know if I was hungry, thirsty, weary or sleepy. I was in a hypervigilant state of caring. My personal needs were nonexistent. In fact, it was very much like those early months with a new baby. I was sleep deprived. I wolfed down my meals as though the baby would wake up at any moment. I showered quickly in the morning and took only the absolute amount of time required to blow dry my hair, dress and put on a touch of make-up.

In hindsight, it was interesting that everyone told me to be sure to take care of myself but no one took me aside and pointed out that this hypervigilant mode of superwoman was not serving the best interests of my body, mind or soul.

If there is any one thing I could have done differently in those months, it would have been to take better care of myself. I would have taken the time to get some sleep, to relieve the stress that was building in my body by enjoying a hot bubble bath now and again. I would have called upon my family and friends to help with Gerry's care or at least asked for them to sit with him more often or take him for a drive while I read a few pages of a book or watched a movie with my daughters. It makes sense to me now. But at the time, self-care was not in my vocabulary nor did I have the trust in my friends or family to take over my responsibilities and do a good job of it.

I wish I had been able to see that I would have been better equipped to handle the day to day situations as they arose by stealing 10 to 15 minutes to renew my spirit through rest, a walk or play time with my children.

You know the stock saying – "If you get sick, you won't do anyone any good." Well, it's true. Unfortunately, we toss this phrase out to people as a way of encouraging them or as a way of demonstrating our concern. But we don't necessarily offer solutions for what the person can do. We may not be helping identify just how the person's well being may be jeopardized by their actions.

Women are notorious for not taking time to care for themselves. Many see it as selfish and a sign of not putting their family first. In some ways, we are shifting this thinking. Today many women – both stay-at-home moms and those working outside the home – take regular time for exercising at the gym, time for personal and professional development and time for massages, pedicures, manicures and hairstyles. The problem is that when you move into the role of primary caregiver, those small luxuries are the first things you toss out the window.

There are sound medical reasons why caregivers should take time for self-care that go beyond the obvious reasons of something you need and deserve. It is well documented that a caregiver's health has increased risks for dementia, Alzheimer's, and can even lead to a shortened life span. Caregiving takes it toll on our lives.

Having said that, it does little good to push people to take time for self-care. It's overwhelming to think of reclaiming 30 minutes in the day to just do something nice for yourself. Besides, if you push caregivers into taking too much time off or engaging in an activity that they have never found enjoyable – albeit relaxing – they will only become frustrated or angry. And if their time away from their loved one is filled with guilt and sadness because they are away – even temporarily – they will not return to their caregiving tasks feeling rested or rejuvenated. It's far better for people to take small breaks and brief interludes of self-care and ease into longer periods of separation. In time, they may choose to leave their loved one overnight or for a weekend and get away for a visit with a friend, attend a retreat, or just enjoy the solitude of being home alone.

Whether you are a service provider, friend, or family member, the following thoughts and tips may be of value to you when encouraging a caregiver to take some time for self-care. The final section is dedicated to caregivers.

Thoughts and Tips

Family and Friends

✓ **Know that it is very difficult for caregivers to be separated from a loved one.** If the injured person is confined to a hospital or rehabilitation center, the caregiver will more likely be interested or persuaded to take a break when the loved one is sleeping or if the facility has an "enforced no visiting time" when the patient is resting.

✓ **Caregivers may not realize they are hypervigilant in caring for their loved one.** Don't confront them as it will only put them in a defensive mode. Instead, gently point out that they are neglecting their own needs for rest and proper nutrition, as well as their physical and spiritual needs.

✓ **Insisting that caregivers take a break for some exercise will likely be met with defiant resistance.** If caregivers had 45 minutes a day for intense aerobics they'd feel like they were on a holiday. They will likely tell you they barely have time to eat, sleep or tend to their personal care. Offering to replace them for a brief 10 minutes while they take a walk around the block won't seem so intense or neglectful to their loved one and a brisk 10 minute walk can do wonders to rejuvenate the body and mind.

✓ **Offer to take over the mundane duties like laundry, washing the floors and cleaning the toilets.** Pick up groceries and cook a few meals and stock the freezer. Caregivers have little time or energy for these tasks. Organize a group to rotate and help out with household tasks. Remember these families' lives are in chaos. If their houses are in chaos, it only compounds the situation.

✓ **Be sensitive to the beliefs, culture and traditions of families.** If you know, for example, that the family attends a church regularly, offer to spell the caregiver off to attend a service. If the caregiver resists, don't push it but instead offer to attend church with any children. It can be quite comforting for the caregiver to know that the children are engaging in some routine activities. Most of all, if the response is "no," ask again next week. As time moves forward, our perspectives change and perhaps the timing will be right later on. Don't wait for caregivers to ask you – it will likely never happen and they probably won't even remember that you offered in the first place.

✓ **Recognize that the energy of caregivers is zapped.** Their spirit may be low and their ability to focus and concentrate may be diminished. They may not even be able to tell you what they need or want to do. It's important to be respectful and not attempt to take over or boss people around. It is okay to try and foresee how you can help and then offer to do that but don't try to take over.

✓ **Don't commit to something you can't do.** If you can't keep up the pace of visiting twice a week, then don't set it up that way. Be honest. If you can give one-half hour once a week or twice a month – offer that and stick to it. Once you gain the trust of the caregiver they will be looking forward to the respite or help. Don't cancel unless it's for a very good reason.

Service Providers/Medical Personnel

✓ **Recognize the need of caregivers to be with their loved one.** Having been told your husband or wife or child is in critical condition and may not live causes the family to re-evaluate and see life very differently. Try to imagine how you would feel in their situation.

✓ **Listen to what people are saying about their loved one.** Chances are you may be doing routine checks but they have been diligently at their loved one's side and may notice or be aware of things you are not. If they feel you are interested in their loved one and that you will genuinely step in for them, they will probably begin to take small breaks.

✓ **Keep foremost in your mind that while this family may be one of dozens of families in your caseload, this is their ONLY family.** They may seem to act like, "It's all about them" but that's because – it *is* all about them! This is the only family they have and they are desperately trying to maintain some control amidst the chaos.

✓ **Families can teach you as much as you can teach them.** Don't approach them with a "god-like" attitude. They are the experts in what is happening to them.

Caregivers

✓ **Keep family and friends informed.** Many people, especially in the early days, will want to know about your loved one's condition and progress. The task of answering telephone calls can be time consuming and exhausting. Some suggestions to help with this are:

1. Set up a voice mailbox through the phone company where you can leave updated messages on a daily basis and where callers can leave you messages. An advantage to this is that you can listen to the messages when you have time and you are feeling up to it.

2. If you use an answering machine – instead of voice mail – change the message daily to give up-to-date information. You can choose not to answer the telephone until you hear who it is and decide if you feel up to talking at that particular moment or not.

3. Enlist a relative or close friend to take calls at their home number for you. You can then schedule a time at your convenience to return the calls.

4. Write one letter that can be photocopied or emailed to friends and family about how the brain injury has affected your loved one and your family. This will help educate them and prepare them for a visit.

✓ **Ask for help.** Your attention and energy will be stretched in many ways. You need to organize, advocate, be a caregiver and perhaps even hold down an outside job. You will need help – don't be afraid to ask. Generally, family and friends want to help – they just don't know what to do. They need to know the best way to help, so make a list of things they can do for you. Some suggestions are: food shopping, caring for other children, cooking meals, checking your home for security and mail, cleaning and laundry, making or canceling appointments, driving or helping with transportation, making phone calls, caring for pets, and staying with you at the hospital.

✓ **Taking 10 minute walks or a 15 minute power nap will re-energize your body, clear your mind and allow your spirit to emerge.** You won't be neglecting your loved one. Instead, you will be ensuring that you can keep up the pace to be a caregiver in the long run.

✓ **Know that brain injury is forever.** Your situation will likely improve over time and with a series of ups and downs over a period of weeks, months or years. Set your pace to go the distance. There are no shortcuts.

✓ **Take inventory of your life.** What were your joys or pleasures prior to this happening? Maybe you don't feel you can take the time you did before, but can you modify any of these activities or break them into small steps so that you can still participate in a meaningful way?

✓ **Take note of how stress is stored in your body or how you react to it.** Do you tend to not eat – or overeat? Do you lean toward using alcohol or medications as a way of helping you cope? If so, consider talking to a professional to obtain some guidance. You will only put yourself at further risk if any of these begin to take hold on your life.

✓ **Is there something that brings you peace?** Tranquil music, meditation, journal writing or quiet time for reflection? Can you carve out some time each day to do this? Take the time. When your loved one is sleeping or has a visitor, sit quietly and listen to music or write. You will be surprised at how just a few minutes each day can build in momentum to restore your spirit.

✓ **Take care of your physical needs.** If you are having trouble sleeping then ask your doctor to give you something mild to help you. There are lots of medications that are useful for temporary situations to help you fall asleep or even to stay asleep if waking up through the night seems to be your problem. Sleep deprivation puts your health at further risk but it also can put the safety of your life or others at risk too. For example, if you drive after putting in an 18 hour day, it is equivalent to driving while under the influence at .05% alcohol. Taking short naps throughout the day is an effective way to offset a shortened night's sleep.

✓ **Try to eat balanced meals.** When you are in shock – which can last for months – you don't necessarily feel like eating. Don't fall into the trap of depending on high doses of caffeine to get you through the day or spiking out on sugar as a means to fuel your body. Poor eating habits over a long time can lead to all kinds of complications like obesity or diabetes to name just a few. It's okay to not want big meals. Eat smaller meals and have a couple of snacks during the day and evening instead. When your friends and family offer to do something to help, enlist one or two of them to make nutritional soups that you can freeze in small portions and reheat in the microwave.

✓ **Take time to feel.** You are going through a major upheaval in your life. Your family roles may have to be adjusted permanently. There can be feelings of sadness, anger, fear and loss. Acknowledge what you feel. Don't suppress it or attempt to sidestep it. These feelings don't just go away if you ignore them. They will manifest in other ways like chemical dependency, destructive relationships, or even disease. If you take time and give yourself permission to feel what is happening, you can move beyond the feelings. It's not to say that you will necessarily "get over" what has happened to you, but you can integrate what has happened and move your life forward in a very positive and meaningful way.

✓ **Don't dismiss professional help.** People often get caught up in thinking they will be in therapy for months or years. You'd be surprised. Most people can garner a new perspective about their situation in just 2 or 3 sessions with a professional. Not everyone needs to see a professional. Somes may benefit from attending a self-help group run by lay people or counselors who have personally experienced a similar situation. And others may find counsel and gain clarity in a therapy group. The point is – don't feel you have to do this alone.

✓ **Connect with a Brain Injury Association or support group in your area.** In the United States, contact the Brain Injury Association of America to obtain a listing for an organization near you. The Family Helpline can be reached by calling 1-800-444-6443 or by email at familyhelpline@biausa.org. To obtain a listing of State Affiliates on the Internet, go to www.biausa.org.

In Canada, contact the Lower Mainland Brain Injury Association at 1-800-510-3221 to obtain a listing of Brain Injury Associations or local support groups in your community.

To Grieve
or Not to Grieve?

Since my husband's death in 1990, I have come to learn that I will grieve his departure from our lives for as long as I live. I have also learned that while his physical death occurred nearly six months after the crash, my children and I were grieving the "death of his personality" during the months he lived. To be honest, I don't know that I can tell you which was more painful.

Certainly to not have him present over the years to watch our children grow up and accomplish many things has been somewhat sad for them and for me. As a couple, we planned (like everyone else) to be together as we grew old, to watch our daughters graduate, to experience thcm falling in love and marry the man of their dreams, and to relish in the glory of being perceived as the best grandparents in the world!

My spiritual beliefs bring comfort in knowing he has walked along side us in our journey. But it is not the same as having him here to talk with, to touch, or to share in our lives on a daily basis. Our lives are void of his perspective and while we strive to honor him in all we do, there remains a deep scar from our family being ripped apart.

Within a very short time of Gerry waking from a coma, I knew he was not the same person. At first the changes were obvious – he acted inappropriately, he talked with a British accent, and he suffered from retrograde amnesia. Not only did he not recognize the people he had close intimate relationships with – like me – but he had no recollection of important events in his life, such as our wedding or his graduation as a police officer.

Over time those memories returned and pieces of the puzzle were put back in place for him. He had a history again, experiences to call upon, and the "who" that we had been as a family unit and all that we had accomplished together once again became the vivid, rich tapestry of his life.

I felt blessed when his memory returned. It had been very painful when he didn't recognize me or even understand what role I played in his life. I think it's fair to say that both Gerry and our children were relieved when his memory returned too.

Ironically, what was initially a godsend (the return of his memory) soon became the very thing that tormented him day in and day out. And in many ways, it tormented me and the girls too. We were acutely aware of the family we had been right up to 8:00 pm on May 19, 1990. And, in an unspoken way, each one of us sensed it was a life that once was - and was never to be again. We just couldn't get back there. In many ways, none of us could put our finger on exactly what was wrong.

Within about six weeks, Gerry looked great. His physical injuries had pretty much healed. He had lost weight and looked younger as a result. But it was more than that. His once crystal blue eyes no longer had a sparkle but instead had a flat hollow look to them. He did not have the same sense of humor as prior to being injured. He lacked self-awareness and did not have the ability to make sound judgments, which meant he continually put himself and others at risk with his actions. He was no longer able to "take charge" with the girls, help out with chores around the house, or even manage his personal care. There was no discussion or planning as a family anymore. He never asked if we needed anything, or if he could do something for us, or even how we were. Everything was about his getting through the day. I don't say that in a spiteful or demeaning way. That was the reality of how we were living. He desperately wanted to be the father and husband he had been prior to the crash – and we wanted him to be too. Every morning, each of us woke with the "silent hope" that today would be just a little more like it used to be.

Gerry tried everyday, but his inability to cope with even the slightest stress in his daily routine or to overcome his depression all worked to sabotage his efforts within hours of his awakening. This in turn meant that all of us would be affected for the day.

At the time, I didn't realize that on top of all the pressures I was trying to juggle – being both mother and father to our children, nurse, advocate and caregiver and financial supporter to the household – I too was depressed and grieving the loss of the man I married. I honestly had no insight into what I was feeling. After all, he was there in flesh and blood standing before me. Even though he had that perpetual "lost soul" look in his eyes, he looked good physically. But there was no doubt he was different. That meant that we as a couple and a family were different too.

Of all the professionals thrust into our lives (doctors, lawyers, physiotherapists, occupational therapists, neurosurgeons, neurologists and psychologists) there wasn't one who broached the topic of grief with us.

In retrospect, I don't believe the grieving process had been acknowledged in traumatic injuries at that time. Certainly, in recent years, the topic has been introduced through support groups and even been presented at brain injury conferences. Nonetheless, by and large, I would have to say that the concept of individuals and families grieving the loss of the lives they had prior to their loved one being brain injured is a relatively new concept. In fact, I regularly hear from workers in the field and family members themselves, that the concept of "grief and loss" being connected to brain injury is met with a somewhat cool reception. When families tell me this, my response is: If someone working with you and your family is not open to the concept of grief and loss in brain injury, then you would be wise to dismiss them and find someone new to work with. I believe they will do you more harm than good.

Part of the problem is that there are still so many misconceptions around grief, bereavement, mourning and loss. It's surprising, I know! We will all experience a "death" of some kind during our lifetime – in fact, none of us will leave this earth without being affected by it. So why is it the least talked about experience and the one we are least prepared for? When something happens to us that involves an "ending" or a "death" in our life, why do we avoid going through the experience, or why do we attempt to prevent someone else from going through it? Fear, I think.

We can experience "death" in a multitude of ways. Sometimes death is physical and sometimes it is not. Our lives can be significantly altered or transformed by "death-like" endings of a job, divorce, friendship, loss of security through financial disaster, or through the loss of our personal identity as when a spouse dies. But there is also another type of death that brings sorrow and pain and that is the death of a personality. This happens when a loved one is debilitated by a disease like Alzheimer's or when life is altered by a catastrophic brain injury.

Generally, it is more common to identify grief and loss with physical death. It's important to acknowledge that the pain and sorrow individuals and families feel when a loved one dies is real, deep and life-altering. You won't have to go far in your own life to find someone who can share with you how life was transformed because of someone's death. Talk to your neighbors, your friends, or your colleagues and they will tell you how they felt when their father or mother died or when their grandparents or a sibling died. The intensity of their feelings will be shaped by what their relationship with the person was like, the circumstance of the person's death, or perhaps even the age of the person.

Scores of citizens around the world have been affected in different ways and on multiple levels by the deaths of complete strangers. For example, the world mourned the death of Princess Diana, and every city, state and country reeled with sorrow when the World Trade Centers in New York City were bombed on September 11, 2001 and over 2,000 innocent individuals lost their lives. These are only two examples. Many people were equally saddened by the deaths of Mother Teresa and Elvis Presley. The point is that when we feel a connection (on whatever level) with someone, we feel pain and sadness when they no longer are a part of our life or we feel deep sympathy and sorrow for the families they have left behind.

What happens though when the mourning is complicated such as in our case, when the family is grieving the "death of a personality" of their father and husband – essentially the family as they once knew it? Is society as tolerant of their perceived loss in this kind of situation? The answer is yes and no.

The *yes* part of this answer comes into play immediately following the injury. Initially, friends and extended family rally around to support the injured person and the immediate family. However, over time that attention begins to wane. To begin with, everyone has a life (children, spouse and job) which will eventually clamor for their attention. You can only give and "be there" for someone for a certain period of time and then your focus naturally turns back to your own life. Otherwise you could jeopardize your own relationships, financial stability or health.

When the situation involves a "life-long" change like a brain injury and especially when the person who is injured experiences significant personality changes, people don't always know how to relate or respond. For example, the social circle of a person with a brain injury who behaves inappropriately or displays significant mood swings often shrinks over time. It isn't that coworkers, buddies or relatives don't care – they do! They just don't understand what's happened and/or how to cope with the changes in the person's personality.

The *no* part to this answer is that society often dismisses people's grief when it is not a physical death or when it's not socially acceptable to mourn that loss (i.e. the family of Timothy McVey – Oklahoma bomber – would not necessarily be supported to publicly mourn his death). This tends to happen as well when someone has been catastrophically injured. Many well-meaning people said things to me after Gerry's accident like, "Well, at least he is alive" or "It could have been worse." Let me declare outright … there were days that I honestly didn't think it "could have been worse." I know they were only trying to help me see the bright side of things, but it didn't do anything to help me resolve or reconcile the deep sense of loss that I was feeling.

I have said throughout this book that I didn't feel like Gerry's wife anymore. It's worth saying it again – *I didn't feel like Gerry's wife anymore.* I wasn't. And he wasn't the husband I had prior to his bike crash either. Furthermore, he no longer had the capacity to father his children the way he had prior to being injured.

The pain and sadness within the walls of our home was immense. He could not be the person he was in any way, shape or form and that meant I could not be the same wife, nor could our daughters be the same children anymore. Instead of playing Barbie dolls and hopscotch, our girls became equal caregivers with me.

I can remember so vividly that I desperately wanted someone – anyone – to validate the sorrow I was feeling because my family was no longer intact.

It's very important that we acknowledge people's grief and we allow them to mourn their loss – including non-physical deaths.

Alan Wolfelt, Ph. D., is the founder and director of the Center for Loss and Life Transition in Fort Collins, Colorado. I met Alan in a round about way through Jeff Nielson, the paramedic who resuscitated Gerry at the crash scene and who, ironically, was the funeral director charged with details of Gerry's funeral. After reviewing an outline for an upcoming book that I am writing on grief and loss, Jeff suggested I send it on to Dr. Wolfelt. I did, and to my pleasant surprise, Dr. Wolfelt contacted me and was very supportive of my work citing that my philosophies were very much in sync with his. Sometime later, I had the pleasure to hear Dr. Wolfelt speak on the topic of complicated mourning. I was riveted by his message and instantly knew that his model of companioning vs. treating people who are grieving was exactly what I had intuitively known and tried to do after Gerry was injured, but did not, or could not put into words.

I have since attended Dr. Wolfelt's Center in Fort Collins to take several courses. By the close of 2003, I will have completed my studies with Dr. Wolfelt and earned a Certificate in Death and Grief Studies through the Center for Loss and Life Transition in conjunction with Colorado State University.

The following will provide you with an overview of Dr. Wolfelt's model of companioning people who are grieving vs. treating people who are grieving.

Five Common Myths about Grieving and Mourning

Contributions by Dr. Alan Wolfelt

Dr. Wolfelt has graciously given permission for me to reprint the *Five Common Myths about Grieving and Mourning* and his *Grieving Person's Bill of Rights*. I have included my comments with the *Five Common Myths about Grieving and Mourning* and will demonstrate how Wolfelt's model fits with families and individuals who have been affected by brain injury. For additional information on the Center for Loss and Life Transition, you are invited to visit Dr. Wolfelt's website at www.centerforloss.com

What are the myths?

Myth 1   Grief and mourning are the same.

Grief and mourning are not the same. Dr. Wolfelt teaches that grieving is our internal response to loss. It's how we feel on the inside – in our hearts, minds and bodies. Mourning is the social response to grief – or grief gone public. It is where we create ceremony and ritual to acknowledge and mark the loss or transformation in our lives.

Myth 2   There is a predictable and orderly stage-like progression to the experience of mourning.

When Dr. Elizabeth Küblor Ross developed the five stages of grief (denial, anger, bargaining, depression and acceptance), it was quickly adopted as the list of feelings that people routinely go through after someone has died or when an individual is faced with a terminal illness. Küblor Ross was correct that these are some of the stages that people may or may not go through. But she did not intend for this list to be taken out of context or interpreted as the list of absolutes that people were expected to feel in a specific order. The reality is that the grieving process is NOT predictable or orderly. If you do go through all five stages you may or may not go through them in the order listed or you may go through some of the stages and again. These are in no particular order.

Myth 3   It is best to move away from the grief.

People tend to back away from the pain of losing someone or something in their life. It's a myth that if you keep busy, or keep a "stiff upper lip" that all will return to normal. It's not true. The only way to heal and begin to bring a sense of normalcy back to your life is to feel what you are feeling and go through the experience.

Myth 4   The goal is to get over your grief.

Again, we tend to want to help people get over their grief. We want them to hurry up and feel better so they are fun to be around again. Here is the truth. You never get over a significant loss. Grief is a lifelong process and one that we integrate into our life but not one that can be dismissed.

Myth 5   Tears are a sign of weakness.

Crying is a healthy way of expressing our feelings. And, it's healthy for everyone – men, women and children. Do it often. Do it freely. And know that you are healing.

Responses to loss

When we are faced with the physical death of a loved one or the ending of something important in our lives, we feel the loss – physically, emotionally and spiritually. For instance, no matter how bad a marriage is when a couple decides to end the relationship through separation or divorce, it can still be very painful and frightening for one person to face life without the other.

Our bodies react to death or death-like experiences with fatigue, lack of appetite and often with an inability to feel joy or happiness.

Our minds react by not being able to concentrate, think things through or by just plain zoning out.

Our spirit reacts by sending us on a search for more meaning or we may feel as though we have a heavy heart or that we have been left with a void in our life.

Our hearts, minds and souls respond to death and grief instinctively. On a conscious level however, we attempt to alter the journey by self-medicating with drugs, overusing alcohol, or by attempting to keep someone or ourselves busy until we get over what has happened. Instead we should be telling others and ourselves to just breathe in and breathe out – just be still. Nothing more.

Let people feel what they are feeling and learn to trust in the process. While they feel those feelings, they will be moving through the feelings and in essence, moving their life forward.

Less than a hundred years ago, everyone in the community knew when a family was going through a loss. Families wore black arm bands and black clothes for one year. A wreath adorned the front door of their home. Neighbors brought baskets of bread and an endless stream of casseroles. Society expected and allowed us to take time to grieve. Today if someone you care about dies, you must qualify as a member of the immediate family before you can be granted a token three day bereavement leave from work.

Over the years, society has adopted a medical-model approach to grieving; one that tends to "treat" people so they can get over their pain. In fact, we want them to do anything but feel their pain!

Intuitively we know what to do to heal when we suffer a loss in our lives. We have no energy to keep up the pace we normally keep. Our body wants to lie down often and we have no desire to eat full meals. In essence, we go into shock and shut down. At times like this we need to stop, feel and just be still.

Companioning vs. treating grief

Dr. Wolfelt's work is based on a growth model of companioning vs. treating people and families who have sustained a loss or death in their lives. To companion an individual or family is to witness their moment-to-moment pain, loss and grief. It is not about being concerned about the outcome of their grieving journey or about leading them through a doorway to resolution. It is about being present during another person's pain. It is about respecting their disorder and confusion – it is about allowing them to be still.

For you and your family to heal and move beyond a loss you need to:
- ✓ Acknowledge the reality of the death or loss
- ✓ Move toward the pain of the loss
- ✓ Remember the person who died (especially if this is a loss of self)
- ✓ Develop a new identity
- ✓ Search for meaning
- ✓ Receive ongoing support from others
- ✓ Know that self-care is critical to being present for others

When you are grieving a loss in your life, remember to have:
- ✓ Patience – there are no rewards for speed – go slowly
- ✓ Heart – be true to your feelings

The Grieving Person's Bill of Rights

by Dr. Alan Wolfelt

You have the right to...
Experience your own unique grief.
Talk about your grief.
Feel a multitude of emotions.
Be tolerant of your physical and emotional limits.
Experience grief attacks
Use ritual.
Embrace your spirituality.
Search for meaning.
Treasure your memories.
Move toward your grief and heal.

I hope you will find strength and courage in these words. You are in a painful time of your life. You have special needs and you have the right to explore your feelings of grief and to mourn your loss.

Remember ... that what you are feeling is not only pain – it is love.